Dermatoscopy

Edited by Paweł Pietkiewicz

Published in London, United Kingdom

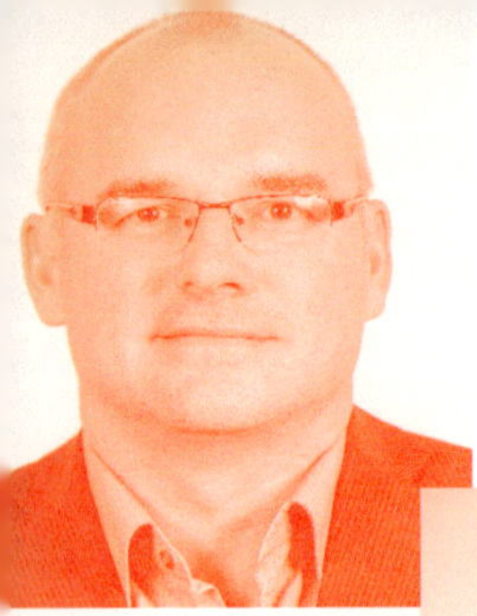
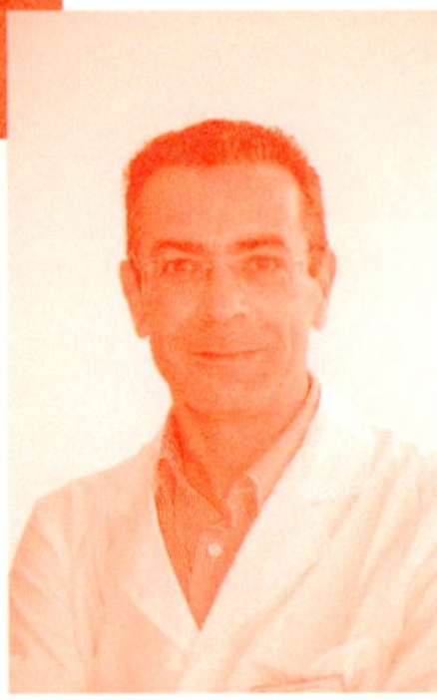
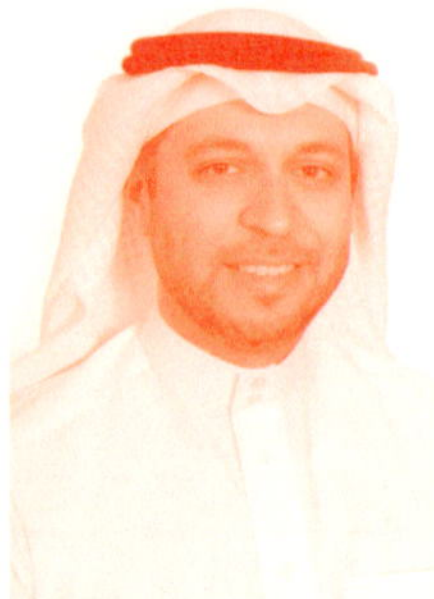
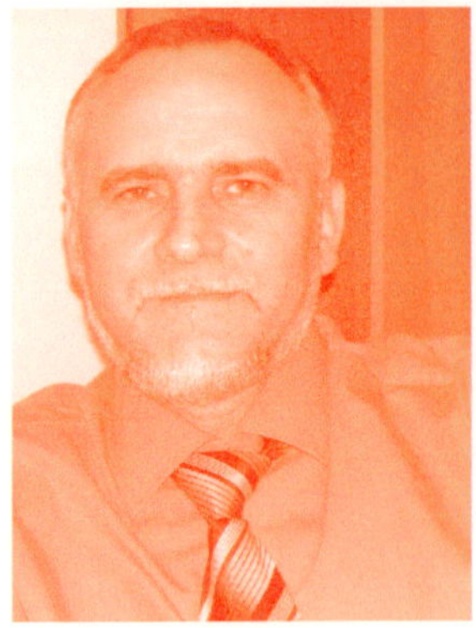
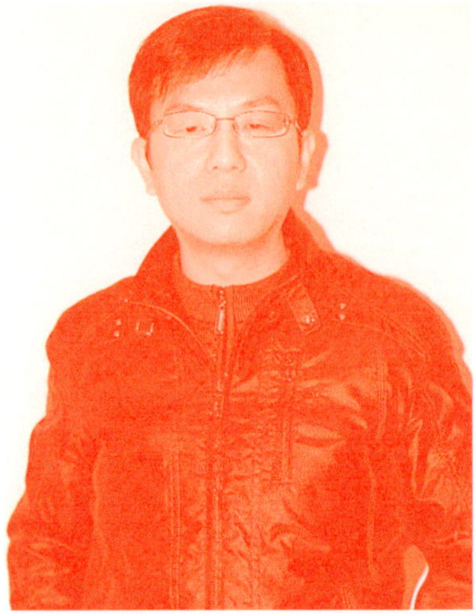
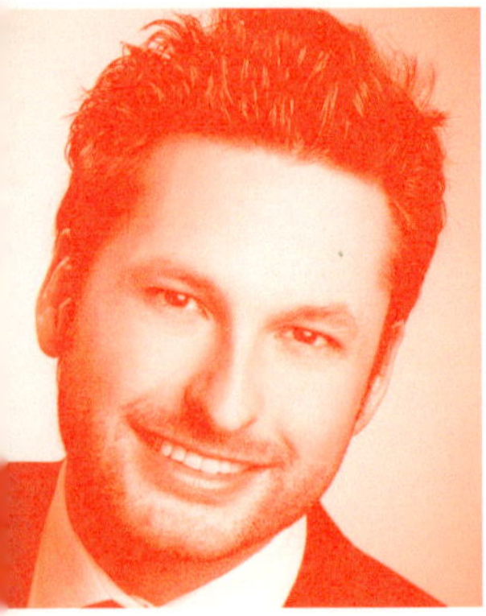
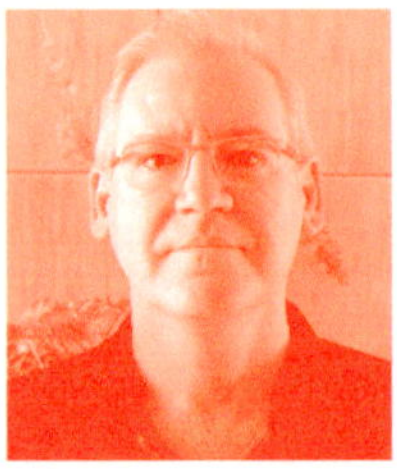

IntechOpen

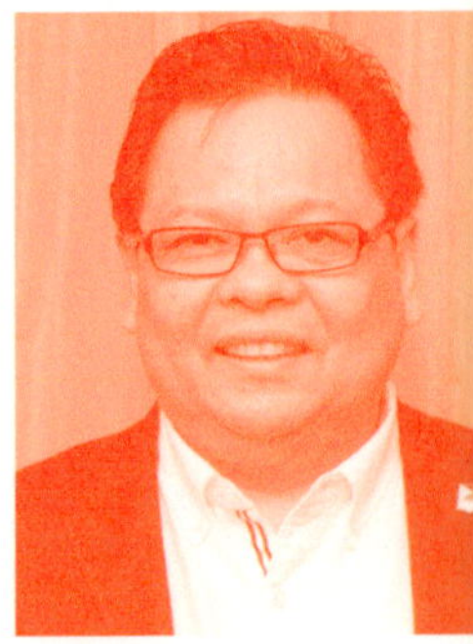
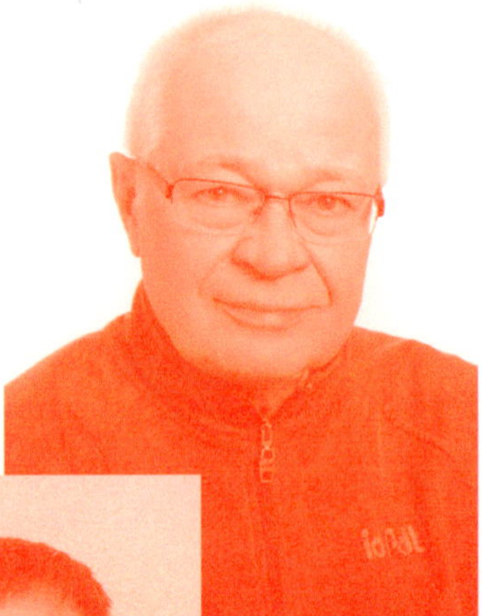
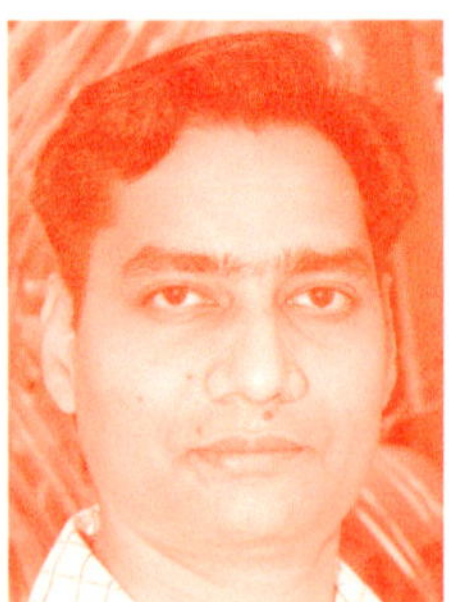
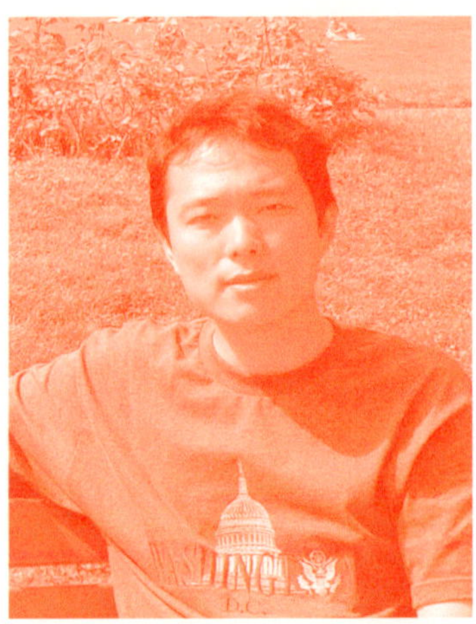
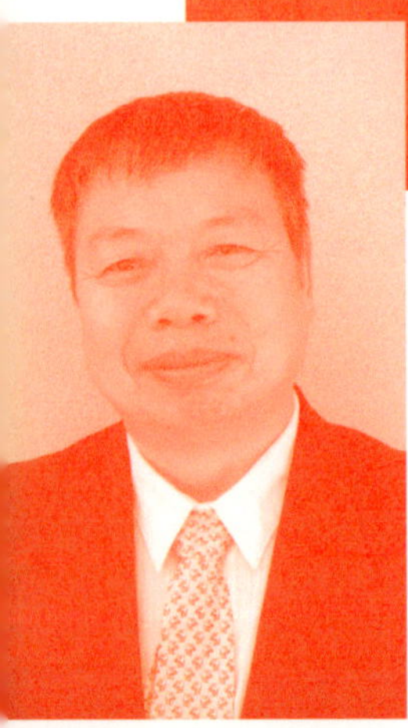
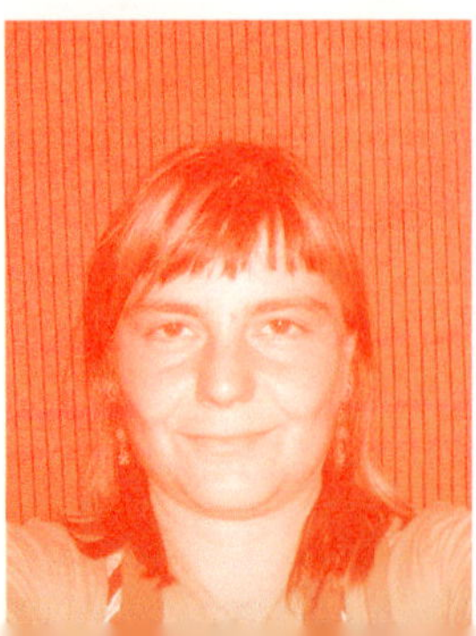

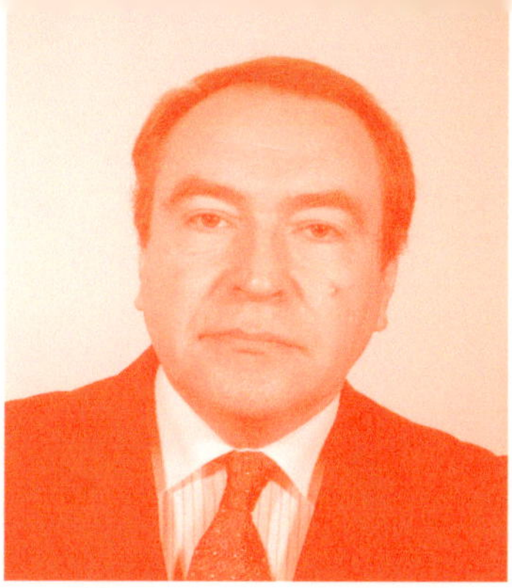
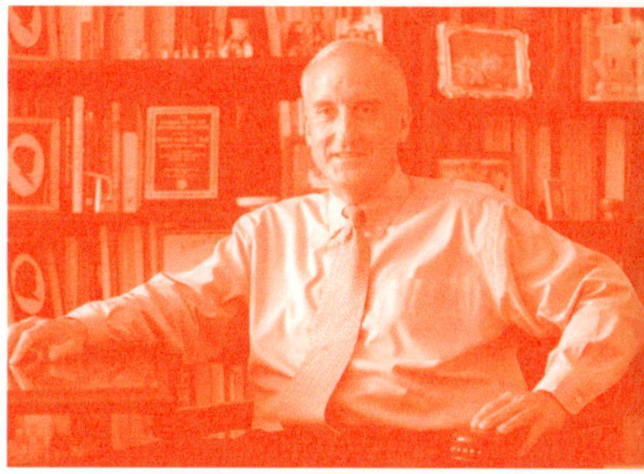
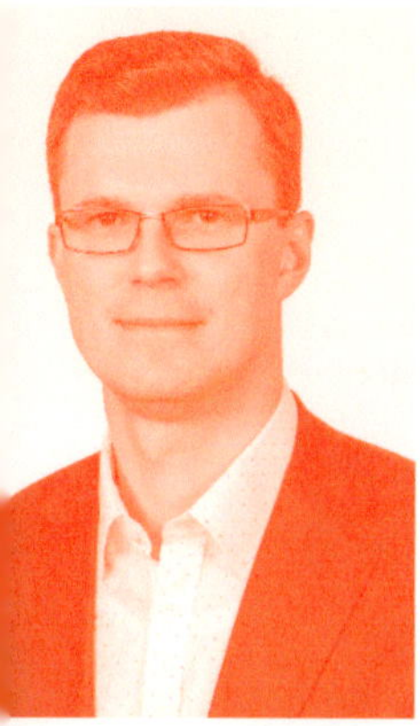
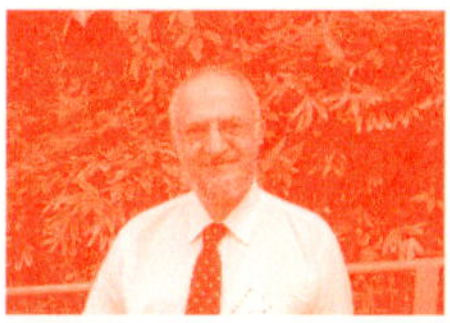
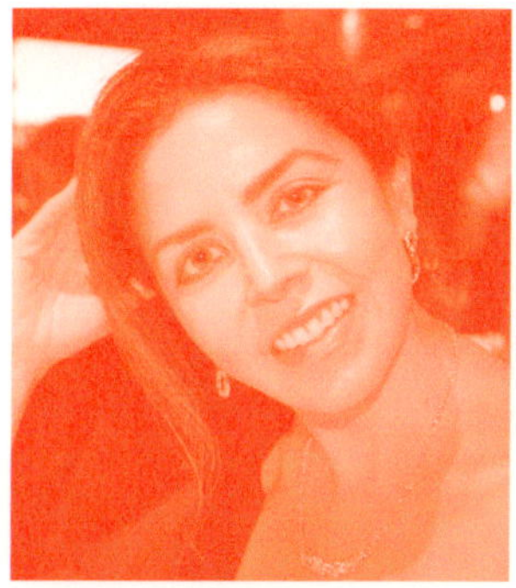

Supporting open minds since 2005

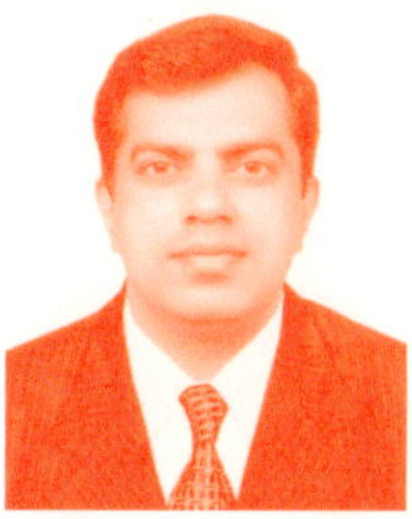
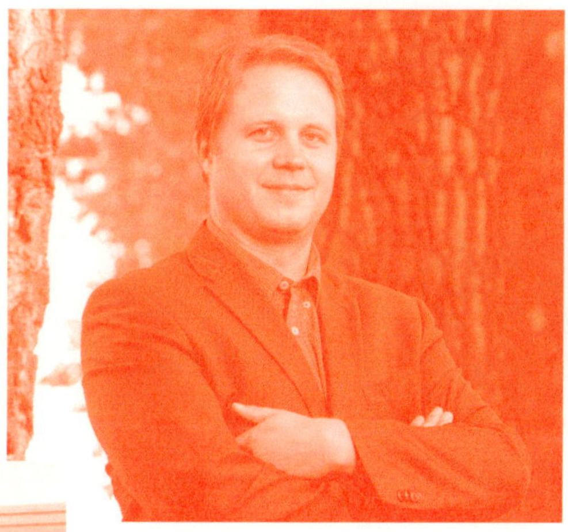
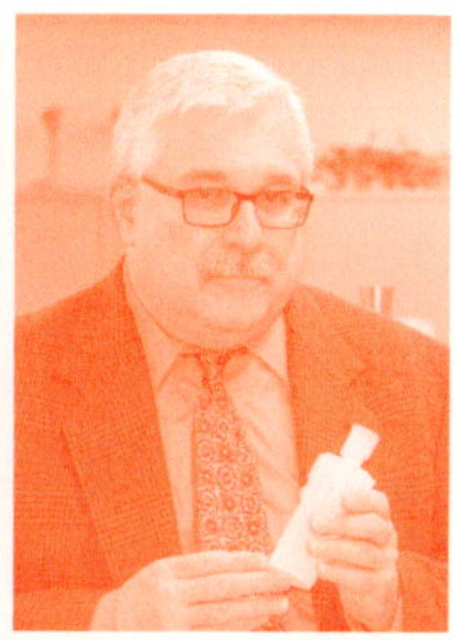
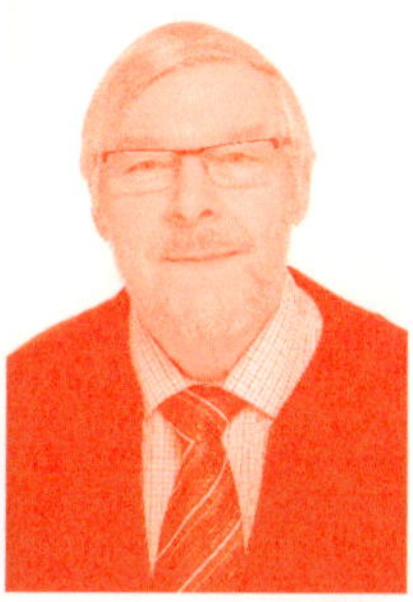
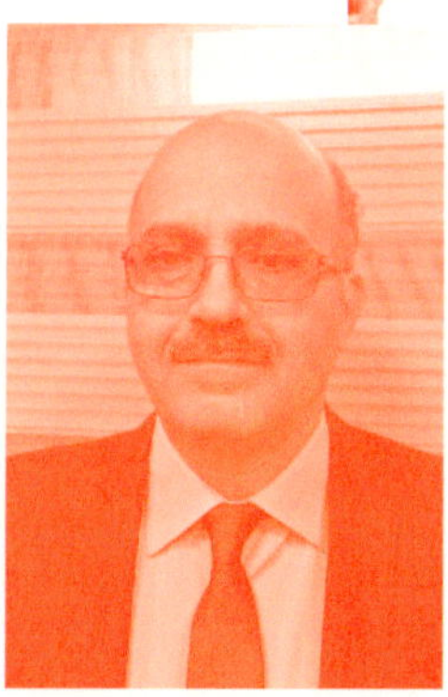
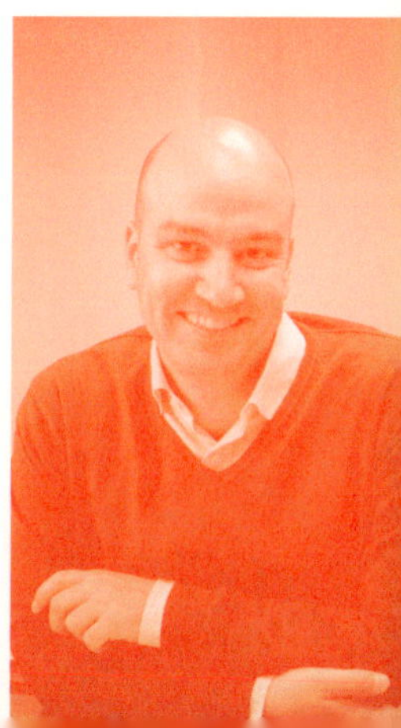
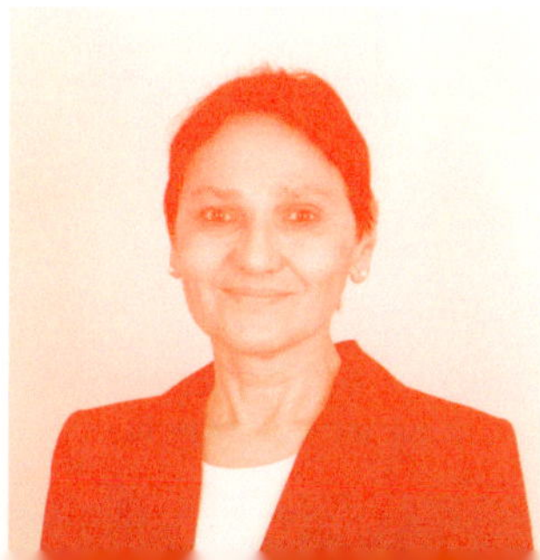

Dermatoscopy
http://dx.doi.org/10.5772/intechopen.95711
Edited by Paweł Pietkiewicz

Contributors
Tubanur Çetinarslan, Aylin Türel Ermertcan, Ece Gökyayla, Alise Balcere, Larisa Prpic-Massari, Nika Hlaca, Tina Zagar, Jelena Stojkovic-Filipovic, Miljan Vlahovic, Walid Al-Zyoud, Dana Erekat, Kinga Adamska, Wojciech Adamski, Paweł Piotr Pietkiewicz

First published in London, United Kingdom, 2022 by IntechOpen
IntechOpen is the global imprint of INTECHOPEN LIMITED, registered in England and Wales, registration number: 11086078, 5 Princes Gate Court, London, SW7 2QJ, United Kingdom
Printed in Croatia

British Library Cataloguing-in-Publication Data
A catalogue record for this book is available from the British Library

Additional hard and PDF copies can be obtained from orders@intechopen.com

Dermatoscopy
Edited by Paweł Pietkiewicz
p. cm.
Print ISBN 978-1-83969-677-0
Online ISBN 978-1-83969-678-7
eBook (PDF) ISBN 978-1-83969-679-4

For EU product safety concerns:
IN TECH d.o.o., Prolaz Marije Krucifikse Kozulić 3, 51000 Rijeka, Croatia, info@intechopen.com or visit our website at intechopen.com.

Meet the editor

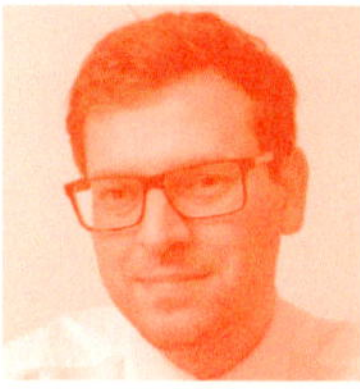

Dr. Paweł Pietkiewicz is a board-certified dermatovenereologist (UEMS-EBDV) working at the Greater Poland Cancer Center. He serves as the president of the Polish Dermatoscopy Group and is a member of the International Dermoscopy Society. His main areas of interest include skin cancer, dermatoscopy, inflammoscopy, and artificial intelligence in dermatology. He is a recipient of the Michael Hornstein Memorial EADV Scholarship (2015), SDF Grant (2015), Euroderm Excellence Grant (2015), SDS Grant (2017), BSPD Grant (2018), EADO Fellowship (2018), Sapienza University of Rome Fellowship (2018), Eli Lilly Grant (2019, 2020), and UCB Scholarship (2021). Dr. Pietkiewicz was a winner of the Dermoscopy Excellence Challenge (2018) and AI Challenges (FotoFinder 2018, 2019; Canfield's DEXI - 2019).

Contents

Preface

Dermatoscopy is a fast, easy-to-learn, low-cost, and non-invasive diagnostic method utilizing the Rayleigh scattering phenomenon to visualize epidermal and subepidermal structures. It has become increasingly popular for allowing visualization of structures that are impossible to see with the naked eye. This book presents comprehensive information on dermatoscopy and its use in detecting skin lesions.

Following the Introductory Section, the second section of this book discusses basal cell carcinoma (BCC) and squamous cell carcinoma (SCC), neoplasms responsible for more than 95% of all skin cancer cases worldwide. Chapter 2 by Prof. Larisa Prpic Massari summarizes the data on epidemiology, genetic background, and the clinical and dermatoscopic presentation of the most common histopathological variants of BCC. In Chapter 3, Dr. Alise Balcere presents an up-to-date review on actinic keratosis (AK) and intraepithelial carcinoma (IEC). This chapter discusses the clinical and histological classification of AK, the SCC progression model, and dermatoscopic clues to AK and IEC.

The third section of this book presents information on melanocytic lesions with a focus on combined nevi, which are common melanoma simulators. In Chapter 4, Prof. Jelena Stojkovic-Filipovic and Miljan Vlahovic define combined nevi and discuss their most common variants and their matching dermatoscopic and histopathologic presentations.

The fourth section of this book focuses on special sites. In Chapter 5, Dr. Wojciech Adamski, an ophthalmologist, and Dr. Kinga Adamska, a dermatologist, present their collection of pigmented lesions affecting the eyelid margin and share their approach to management.

The fifth section includes two miscellaneous chapters. Chapter 6 by Dr. Çetinarslan Tubanur, Dr. Ece Gökyayla, and Prof. Aylin Türel Ermertcan presents the authors' research on inflammoscopy of palmoplantar dermatoses. Rich descriptions of dermatoscopic clues of psoriasis, eczema, lichen planus, and lichen nitidus, a wide range of keratodermas, and fungal and bacterial infectious diseases (including syphilis) are the best examples of where dermatoscopy can be applied. Finally, Chapter 7 by Dr. Walid Al-Zyoud and Dr. Dana Erekat summarizes the precautions taken in the dermatological office during the COVID pandemic. The chapter stratifies procedures into risk groups and advises on how to safely manage patients, including those requiring skin checkups.

I wish to express my gratitude to all the authors for their contributions and IntechOpen for their support and commitment to the world of open-access literature.

Paweł Pietkiewicz
General and Oncological Surgery Clinic I,
Greater Poland Cancer Center,
Poznań, Poland

Section 1

Introduction

Chapter 1

Introductory Chapter: Dermatoscopy

Paweł Pietkiewicz

1. Introduction

Although dermatoscopy was born as epiluminiscence microscopy many decades ago, it still develops, and hundreds of new papers are being published each year in scientific journals on new discoveries, significance of particular structures, and new applications. Dermatoscopy is no longer just a skin cancer screening technique, but can be employed to a wide variety of non-neoplastic conditions: trichoscopy for the diseases of hair and scalp, inflammoscopy for inflammatory skin diseases, mucoscopy for mucous membranes, onychoscopy for the diseases of nail apparatus, infectoscopy for identification of inflammatory diseases, endomodermatoscopy for skin parasitoses, and even dentoscopy for examining the teeth [1–3]. The systematization of the terminology in dermatoscopy and inflammoscopy terminology made the method more accessible for the beginners [4, 5].

2. The scope of dermatoscope

We are living in the era of Internet, smartphones, and artificial intelligence (AI)-driven networks that shape our practices and everyday environment to make it seemingly more convenient and remote, and COVID pandemic accelerated this process even more. In this chase, we are gradually losing the direct contact with our patients, which might lead to delayed or imprecise diagnosis of skin conditions. While taking advantage of what the modern technology provides us with, we should keep in mind that the simplest and direct examination, including taking medical history, visual inspection, and palpation, should still remain a gold standard. Dermatoscope is fast to apply and inexpensive auxiliary tool that complements physical examination and gives a better insight into the true nature of the inspected lesion. Nowadays, in many situations, dermatoscopists are able to diagnose certain diseases or predict a number of details commonly provided in pathology reports without actually taking a biopsy. Dermatoscopes proved to be useful in multispecialty settings. These can be used by dermatologists, oncologists, surgeons, general practitioners, radiotherapists, urologists, hematologists, pathologists, and many more. Being able to identify dermatoscopic structures can be the first step into pattern analysis and learning dermatoscopy-pathology correlations [6–8]. Currently, it is possible to assess tumor margins better than with a naked eye, which lowers the costs of treatment and lowers the risk of recurrence after radiotherapy and skin surgery, especially in Mohs micrographic surgery [9–14]. Particular structures, such as pigmented clods, or vascular clues, can be predictors of more invasive basal and squamous cell carcinomas (BCC, SCC) [15–20]. Consequently, it has an impact on planning the management (namely choosing between the surgery, topical treatment, radiotherapy, or photodynamic therapy) or monitoring its efficacy [21–24].

Dermatoscopy always provides meaningful information. It may either confirm or rule out initial clinical diagnosis or point out to the other diagnosis that was not considered initially, especially inflammatory skin diseases. Even if the lesion turns out to be mysterious to the eye of dermatoscopist, dermatoscopy may exclude some of the diagnoses and lead to change in the diagnostic plan and management, influencing the decisive process (e.g., rapid biopsy)and saving the patient from the consequences of diagnostic pitfall, unnecessary expenses for non-optimal therapy and its side effects, lost time till the final diagnosis, unnecessary stress and suffering, and in some cases, also patient's life/health from disease progression.

When combined with a device to capture images (smartphone, single-lens reflex camera, compact camera, or more convenient professional video dermatoscope) it proves to give additional info on already excised lesions. With a digitized image, physician is able to verify his initial diagnosis and reconsult the slides with the pathologist in order to avoid medical errors if the initial diagnosis does not match the report. It enables the identification of cases of mismatched specimens, misdiagnosis, or invalid tumor subtype. Also, based on the significance of the spectrum of colors seen in dermatoscopy, it is possible to detect underestimated Breslow thickness, as gray and blue colors mark the distribution of melanin in papillary and reticular dermis [25]. This process of confronting certain digitized features with the pathology can be called retroscopy, which is also a useful method to learn the morphology-histology correlations. Digital dermatoscopy or monitoroscopy can also be used for monitoring inflammatory skin diseases, predicting the therapeutic outcomes and resistance/susceptibility to certain therapies [26, 27]. AI is being increasingly implemented in all areas of healthcare. AI-assisted wide area digital dermatoscopy is a method enabling to combine multiple separate dermatoscopic images of the same large skin lesion into one map to enable precise assessment of structures and delineation [28–30]. Assessing the borders in melanoma is crucial for radical excision. In some lesions, this border is vague, but dermatoscopy with wavelengths close to ultraviolet light is able to enhance this process [31]. Another computer-assisted add-on to dermatoscopy and inflammoscopy is skin parameter map obtained with multispectral dermatoscopy [32–34]. Pattern recognition algorithms may have a particularly important role in the future development of digital dermatoscopy, supporting the diagnostic process and assisting the management, especially for non-experts [35]. This applies not only to AI-assisted assessment of dermatoscopic images but also photographs obtained with total body photography (TBP) [36–40]. Combining sequential TBP with the sequential digital dermatoscopy imaging increases the accuracy of detection of smaller, less invasive melanomas but also reduces the number of unnecessary surgical procedures [41]. As handheld dermatoscopy is cost-effective, easy to apply and learn, it is this diagnostic technique that should serve as a basic auxiliary device in skin cancer screening.

Author details

Paweł Pietkiewicz
General and Oncological Surgery Clinic I, Greater Poland Cancer Center,
Poznań, Poland

*Address all correspondence to: p.pietkiewicz@mp.pl

References

[1] Micali G, Lacarrubba F. The expanding use of dermatoscopy. Dermatologic Clinics. 2018;**36**(4):xv

[2] Verzì AE, Lacarrubba F, Dinotta F, Micali G. Dermatoscopy of parasitic and infectious disorders. Dermatologic Clinics. 2018;**36**(4):349-358

[3] Jha A, Pathak J, Sonthalia S, Keshavmurthy V. Use of polarized dermoscopy in the evaluation of congenital erythropoietic porphyria. Clinical and Experimental Dermatology. 2021;**46**(3):556-557

[4] Kittler H, Marghoob AA, Argenziano G, Carrera C, Curiel-Lewandrowski C, Hofmann-Wellenhof R, et al. Standardization of terminology in dermoscopy/dermatoscopy: Results of the third consensus conference of the International Society of Dermoscopy. Journal of the American Academy of Dermatology. 2016;**74**(6):1093-1106

[5] Errichetti E, Zalaudek I, Kittler H, Apalla Z, Argenziano G, Bakos R, et al. Standardization of dermoscopic terminology and basic dermoscopic parameters to evaluate in general dermatology (non-neoplastic dermatoses): An expert consensus on behalf of the international Dermoscopy society. The British Journal of Dermatology. 2020;**182**(2):454-467

[6] Russo T, Piccolo V, Ferrara G, Agozzino M, Alfano R, Longo C, et al. Dermoscopy pathology correlation in melanoma. The Journal of Dermatology. 2017;**44**(5):507-514

[7] Yélamos O, Braun RP, Liopyris K, Wolner ZJ, Kerl K, Gerami P, et al. Dermoscopy and dermatopathology correlates of cutaneous neoplasms. Journal of the American Academy of Dermatology. 2019;**80**(2):341-363

[8] Kasuya A, Aoshima M, Fukuchi K, Shimauchi T, Fujiyama T, Tokura Y. An intuitive explanation of dermoscopic structures by digitally reconstructed pathological horizontal top-down view images. Scientific Reports. 2019;**9**:19875

[9] Suzuki HS, Serafini SZ, Sato MS. Utility of dermoscopy for demarcation of surgical margins in Mohs micrographic surgery. Anais Brasileiros de Dermatologia. 2014;**89**(1):38-43

[10] Ballester Sánchez R, Pons Llanas O, Pérez Calatayud J, Botella ER. Dermoscopy margin delineation in radiotherapy planning for superficial or nodular basal cell carcinoma. The British Journal of Dermatology. 2015;**172**(4):1162-1163

[11] Shin K, Kim H-J, Ko H-C, Kim B-S, Kim M-B, Kim H-S. Dermoscopy-guided Mohs micrographic surgery in post-laser basal cell carcinomas: Is dermoscopy helpful for demarcation of the surgical margin? Journal of Dermatological Treatment. 2022;**33**(1):433-436

[12] Litaiem N, Karray M, Jones M, Rammeh S, Zeglaoui F. Effectiveness of dermoscopy in the demarcation of surgical margins in slow Mohs surgery. Dermatologic Therapy. 2020;**33**(6): e14196

[13] Carducci M, Bozzetti M, De Marco G, Foscolo AM, Betti R. Usefulness of margin detection by digital dermoscopy in the traditional surgical excision of basal cell carcinomas of the head and neck including infiltrative/morpheaform type. The Journal of Dermatology. 2012;**39**(4):326-330

[14] Carducci M, Bozzetti M, Foscolo AM, Betti R. Margin detection using digital dermatoscopy improves the performance of traditional surgical

excision of basal cell carcinomas of the head and neck. Dermatologic Surgery. 2011;**37**(2):280-285

[15] Apalla Z, Lallas A, Tzellos T, Sidiropoulos T, Lefaki I, Trakatelli M, et al. Applicability of dermoscopy for evaluation of patients' response to nonablative therapies for the treatment of superficial basal cell carcinoma. The British Journal of Dermatology. 2014;**170**(4):809-815

[16] Lallas A, Argenziano G, Kyrgidis A, Apalla Z, Moscarella E, Longo C, et al. Dermoscopy uncovers clinically undetectable pigmentation in basal cell carcinoma. The British Journal of Dermatology. 2014;**170**(1):192-195

[17] Ayhan E, Ucmak D, Akkurt Z. Vascular structures in dermoscopy. Anais Brasileiros de Dermatologia. 2015;**90**(4):545-553

[18] Urech M, Kyrgidis A, Argenziano G, Reggiani C, Moscarella E, Longo C, et al. Dermoscopic ulceration is a predictor of basal cell carcinoma response to Imiquimod: A retrospective study. Acta Dermato-Venereologica. 2017;**97**(1): 117-119

[19] Kato J, Horimoto K, Sato S, Minowa T, Uhara H. Dermoscopy of melanoma and non-melanoma skin cancers. Frontiers in Medicine. 2019;**6**:180. DOI: 10.3389/fmed.2019.00180

[20] Álvarez-Salafranca M, Ara M, Zaballos P. Dermoscopy in basal cell carcinoma: An updated review. Actas Dermo-Sifiliográficas Engl Ed. 2021;**112**(4):330-338

[21] Husein-ElAhmed H, Fernandez-Pugnaire MA. Dermatoscopy-guided therapy of pigmented basal cell carcinoma with imiquimod. Anais Brasileiros de Dermatologia. 2016;**91**(6):764-769

[22] Mainetti C, Guillod C, Leoni-Parvex S. Successful treatment of relapsing Bowen's disease with Ingenol Mebutate: The use of Dermoscopy to monitor the therapeutic response. Dermatol Basel Switz. 2016;**232** (Suppl. 1):9-13

[23] Diluvio L, Bavetta M, Di Prete M, Orlandi A, Bianchi L, Campione E. Dermoscopic monitoring of efficacy of ingenol mebutate in the treatment of pigmented and non-pigmented basal cell carcinomas. Dermatologic Therapy. 2017;**30**(1):e12438

[24] Krzysztofiak T, Kamińska-Winciorek G, Tukiendorf A, Suchorzepka M, Wojcieszek P. Basal cell carcinoma treated with high dose rate (HDR) brachytherapy-early evaluation of clinical and Dermoscopic patterns during irradiation. Cancers. 2021;**13**(20):5188

[25] Colors—Dermoscopedia. Dermoscopedia.org. 2022. Available from: https://dermoscopedia.org/Colors

[26] Vos MHE, Nguyen KP, Van Erp PEJ, Van de Kerkhof PCM, Driessen RJB, Peppelman M. The value of (video) dermoscopy in the diagnosis and monitoring of common inflammatory skin diseases: A systematic review. European Journal of Dermatology. 2018;**28**(5):575-596

[27] Errichetti E. Dermoscopy in monitoring and predicting therapeutic response in general dermatology (non-Tumoral dermatoses): An up-to-date overview. Dermatologic Therapy. 2020;**10**(6):1199-1214

[28] Dellatorre G, Gadens GA. Wide area digital dermoscopy. Journal of the American Academy of Dermatology. 2019;**80**(6):e153

[29] Dellatorre G, Gadens GA. Wide area digital dermoscopy applied to basal cell

carcinoma. Anais Brasileiros de Dermatologia. 2020;**95**(3):379-382

[30] Gadens GA, Dellatorre G. Wide area digital Dermoscopy for congenital melanocytic nevi: Report of 3 cases. Dermatology Practical & Conceptual. 2020;**10**(1):e2020023

[31] Sano T, Minagawa A, Suzuki R, Koga H, Okuyama R. Dermoscopy with near-ultraviolet light highlights the demarcation of melanin distribution in cutaneous melanoma. Journal of the American Academy of Dermatology. 2021;**84**(1):e23-e24

[32] Janssen L, Mylle S, Van Kelst S, De Smedt J, Diricx B, Kimpe T, et al. Enhanced visualization of blood and pigment in multispectral skin dermoscopy. Skin Research and Technology. 2020;**26**(5):708-712

[33] Kaliyadan F, Jayasree P, Kuruvilla J, Errichetti E, Lallas A. The use of blue light, multispectral dermoscopy in vitiligo: A pilot study. Skin Research and Technology. 2020;**26**(4):612-614

[34] Nirmal B. Utility of blue light in Dermoscopy for diagnosing stable lesions in vitiligo. Dermatology Practical & Conceptual. 2021;**11**(1):e2021141

[35] Das K, Cockerell CJ, Patil A, Pietkiewicz P, Giulini M, Grabbe S, et al. Machine learning and its application in skin Cancer. International Journal of Environmental Research and Public Health. 2021;**18**(24):13409

[36] Korotkov K, Quintana J, Puig S, Malvehy J, Garcia R. A new total body scanning system for automatic change detection in multiple pigmented skin lesions. IEEE Transactions on Medical Imaging. 2015;**34**(1):317-338

[37] Tschandl P. Sequential digital dermatoscopic imaging of patients with multiple atypical nevi. Dermatology Practical & Conceptual. 2018;**8**(3):231-237

[38] Hornung A, Steeb T, Wessely A, Brinker TJ, Breakell T, Erdmann M, et al. The value of Total body photography for the early detection of melanoma: A systematic review. International Journal of Environmental Research and Public Health. 2021;**18**(4):1726

[39] Strzelecki MH, Strąkowska M, Kozłowski M, Urbańczyk T, Wielowieyska-Szybińska D, Kociołek M. Skin lesion detection algorithms in whole body images. Sensors. 2021;**21**(19):6639

[40] Grochulska K, Betz-Stablein B, Rutjes C, Chiu FP-C, Menzies SW, Soyer HP, et al. The additive value of 3D Total body imaging for sequential monitoring of skin lesions: A case series. Dermatol Basel Switz. 2022;**238**(1):12-17

[41] Deinlein T, Michor C, Hofmann-Wellenhof R, Schmid-Zalaudek K, Fink-Puches R. The importance of total-body photography and sequential digital dermatoscopy for monitoring patients at increased melanoma risk. Journal der Deutschen Dermatologischen Gesellschaft. 2020;**18**(7):692-697

Section 2

Skin Cancer

Chapter 2

Dermatoscopic Features of Basal Cell Carcinoma

Tina Zagar, Nika Hlaca and Larisa Prpic-Massari

Abstract

Basal cell carcinoma is the most common type of non-melanoma skin cancers, frequently observed in fair-skinned individuals. The major risk factors for developing basal cell carcinoma are environmental exposures, phenotypic and genetic traits, and immunosuppression. The diagnosis of basal cell carcinoma is based upon clinical examination and dermatoscopy findings and finally confirmed by histopathological analysis. There are five main clinicopathologic types of basal cell carcinoma, specifically, superficial, nodular, pigmented, morpheaform, and fibroepithelial variant. The dermatoscopic feature of all BCC is the absence of a pigment network. Dermatoscopy structures are further classified as vascular, pigment-related, and non-vascular/non-pigment-related structures. Vascular structures include arborizing vessels and short fine telangiectasias, while pigmented structures comprise maple leaf-like areas, spoke-wheel areas, multiple blue-gray globules, in-focus dots, and concentric structures. Additional structures such as ulcerations, multiple small erosions, multiple aggregated yellow-white globules, shiny white-red structureless areas, and white streaks are considered non-vascular/non-pigmented structures. As treatment options highly depend on the type of BCC, dermatoscopy is of great value in management strategy, assessment of margins, and evaluation of response to non-ablative therapies.

Keywords: algorithms, dermatoscopy, disease management, carcinoma, basal cell, carcinoma, basal cell/diagnosis, skin neoplasms

1. Introduction

Basal cell carcinoma (BCC) is the most common type of non-melanoma skin cancers (NMSCs), most frequently observed in fair-skinned individuals. BCCs originate from the pluripotent cells of the bulge region of the hair shaft and the interfollicular epidermis. Even though BCCs rarely metastasize, they are locally invasive and destructive, and thus if not treated on time, present a therapeutic challenge. There are five main clinicopathologic types of BCC, specifically, superficial, nodular, pigmented, morpheaform, and fibroepithelial (also familiar as fibroepithelioma of Pinkus) [1].

Regarding epidemiology, the incidence of BCC correlates well with geographic location, with the southern hemisphere and regions closer to the equator having higher incidence. The average amount of annual exposure to ultraviolet radiation (UVR) has insignificant correlation with the incidence of BCCs. Additionally, fair skin phototypes and increasing age are also well correlated with the incidence of

BCC [1, 2]. The median age for acquiring BCC is 68. However, the development of BCC is mostly related to skin color, with white populations being particularly prone to the development of BCC. Moreover, men have a higher risk for acquiring BCC than women, although the rise in BCC among younger women has been noted lately. According to the American Cancer Society, currently, the incidence of BCCs is on the rise by more than 10% per year in the United States. Similar increases in incidence have been observed worldwide over the last two decades [3, 4].

The risk factors for developing BCC are environmental exposures, phenotypic characteristics, genetic traits, and immunosuppression. UVR is the most significant risk factor, particularly intermittent intense episodes of UV exposure and sunburns early in life [4, 5]. Among phenotypic traits, fair skin pigmentation, light hair and eye color, and poor tanning ability are the most common risk factors for BCC [5]. Furthermore, indoor tanning usage, chronic immunosuppression, and to a certain degree long-term photochemotherapy (PUVA) as well as ionizing radiation influence the risk for BCC development [6–8]. Additionally, chronic immunosuppression may increase the risk for BCC [9]. Some inherited diseases such as nevoid basal cell carcinoma syndrome (NBCCS) or Gorlin-Goltz syndrome, xeroderma pigmentosum, Bazex-Dupré-Christol syndrome, Rombo syndrome, and oculocutaneous albinism (OCA) carry a great risk for developing BCC at an early age [10, 11]. Specific gene polymorphisms in regions responsible for pigmentary traits, such as melanocortin-1 receptor (MC1R), the human homolog of agouti-signaling protein (ASIP), and tyrosinase (TYR), are additionally associated with an increased risk for BCC [12].

Pathogenetically, UVR induces mutations in several tumor suppressor genes and proto-oncogenes that consequently lead to BCC formation [13, 14]. Mutations in genes causing hyperactivation of the hedgehog (HH) protein family pathway, including PTCH1 receptor, SMO signal transducer, and GLI transcription factors, are strongly associated with BCC development [15, 16]. Furthermore, the TP53 tumor suppressor gene is also linked to BCC formation. The PTCH1 and TP53 are considered UV signature mutations due to the strong association with UVR-induced mutagenesis [13, 16].

Almost 70% of BCCs arise on the face and 15% on the trunk, while they rarely develop in the genital area [17]. The diagnosis of BCC is based upon clinical examination and dermatoscopy findings and finally confirmed by histopathological analysis. Since dermatoscopic features of BCC strongly assist the clinical diagnosis of BCC, clinicians must be familiar with typical dermatoscopic findings of various subtypes of BCC [17–19].

2. Dermatoscopy of basal cell carcinoma

Dermatoscopy or epiluminescence microscopy is a widely used tool that increases BCC detection accuracy and distinguishes BCC subtypes. Dermatoscopy features of BCC are classified into three main categories: vascular, pigment-related, and non-vascular/non-pigment-related. Vascular structures include arborizing vessels and short fine telangiectasias. Pigment-related structures consist of maple-leaf-like areas, spoke-wheel areas, multiple blue-gray globules (ovoid nests), in-focus dots (peppering/buckshot scatter), and concentric structures. Structures such as ulcerations, multiple minor erosions, shiny white blotches and strands, red structureless areas, and multiple aggregated yellow-white globules are classified as non-vascular/non-pigmented structures [20].

The most significant vascular dermatoscopic feature is arborizing vessels. More than three decades ago, arborizing vessels were described as the main feature of BCC, with high diagnostic accuracy and predictive value of over 90% [21]. However, arborizing vessels are not limited to BCC but to any fast-growing lesions such as cysts and tumors, including benign skin tumors.

Various attempts to categorize dermatoscopic features for particular BCC subtypes have been described. Most of the studies focus on the vascular pattern in different forms of BCC. As mentioned before, besides the role in diagnosing BCC, dermatoscopy is of great value in management strategy, evaluation of response to non-ablative therapies, and margin detection before surgical excision. Regarding the management strategy of treatment, the first step is to distinguish between superficial and non-superficial BCC as it determines further management decision, with non-surgical treatments considered the first-line option for sBCC, while surgical excision being the standard for nodular BCC (nBCC) and Mohs micrographic surgery representing optimal choice for more invasive infiltrative forms of BCC [22, 23]. Superficial BCC is characterized by an optimal response to non-ablative therapies, such as imiquimod and photodynamic therapy (PDT). The authors Urech et al. reveal that dermatoscopic findings of erosions or ulcerations strongly predict a favorable response to imiquimod [24]. The pigment-related structures can act as a competitive light-absorbing factor, significantly reducing the response rate of the tumor to PDT. This observation leads to the exclusion of PDT as a treatment option in the presence of pigmented features [25]. In monitoring the outcome of non-ablative therapeutic modalities, dermatoscopic disappearance of pigmented structures, ulceration, and arborizing telangiectasias are indicators of complete tumor clearance.

Further monitoring is recommended to recognize early post-treatment reappearance of BCC-specific structures. However, the detection of white or red structureless areas and superficial fine telangiectasia does not provide explicit information on the possible presence of residual disease since these features might also appear as a result of treatment-induced skin atrophy [26].

In the non-superficial BCC, dermatoscopy is used in presurgical excision margins marking since it can detect a sub-clinical tumor expansion by revealing disease-related features in peripheral areas of clinically healthy skin.

3. Dermatoscopy of various BCC subtypes

3.1 Dermatoscopy of nodular basal cell carcinoma

Nodular BCC clinically manifests as a flesh-colored papule or nodule with a smooth surface typically located in the face region (**Figure 1A–C**). This subtype of BCCs is the most common and comprises approximately 60–80% of all cases of BCCs [1, 22, 27]. NBCCs usually have a pearly appearance and visible arborizing telangiectasias, while their border is raised compared to the central part of the lesion. This elevated rolled border is one of the critical clues to diagnosis. Additional clinical feature of nodular BCC is ulceration, hence the terms "rodent ulcer" or "phagedenic ulcer" for describing the ulcerating forms of nBCC. In contrast to sBCC, which often emerges on the trunk, nBCCs usually arise in the head and neck area, especially on the cheeks, nose, nasolabial folds, forehead, and eyelids, although they may develop in any hair-bearing area of the skin [1, 2, 22, 28]. The clinical differential diagnosis of non-ulcerated nBCC lesions includes adnexal neoplasms, fibrous papules, intradermal melanocytic nevi, amelanotic melanoma, sarcoidosis, cutaneous tuberculosis, and foreign body granulomas. Regarding ulcerating nBCC, squamous cell carcinoma (SCC) and keratoacanthomas are potential differential diagnoses [29].

NBCC is considered low-risk BCC; hence, standard surgical excision with 4-mm clinical margins with postoperative margin evaluation or electrodessication and

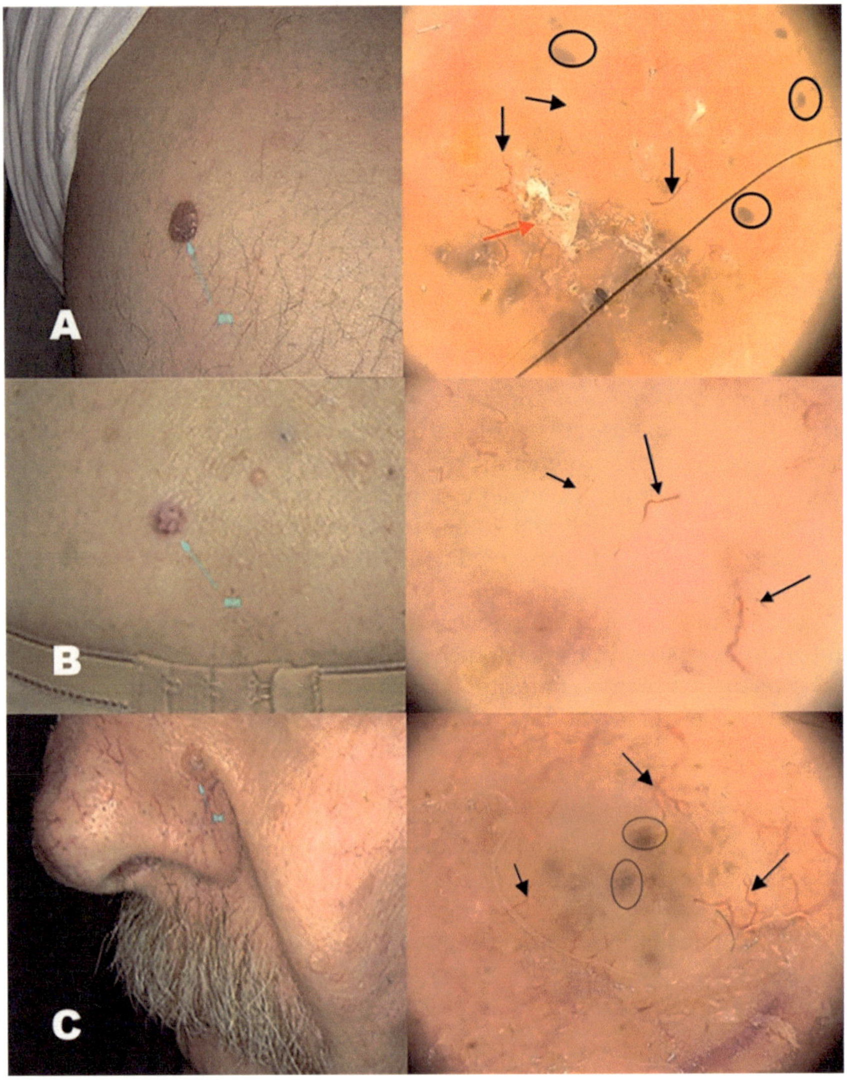

Figure 1.
(A) Left: nodular BCC clinically presented as a pink-colored nodule with a smooth surface. Right: dermatoscopy revealed small arborizing vessels (black arrows), blue-gray globules (circle), and scale due to ulceration (red arrow). (B) Left: nodular BCC may clinically manifest as a growing pink nodule. Right: the hallmark of nodular BCC is arborizing vessels. Be careful, vessels like this may blanch out if you press down hard on the lesion. (C) Left: skin-colored papule on the nose of the patient. Right: arborizing vessels identifiable as larger bright red stem vessels that branch into thinner branches (arrows) and gray-brown ovoid nests (square) are the most distinguishable features of nodular BCC.

curettage (EDC) are the two available treatment options according to the National Comprehensive Cancer Network Clinical Practice Guidelines in Oncology (NCCN Guidelines). EDC is an alternative therapeutic modality for patients who may not tolerate surgery or prefer this non-surgical treatment option [23].

Dermatoscopy findings of nBCC include arborizing vessels, large blue-gray ovoid nests, multiple blue-gray dots/globules, and ulcerations (**Figure 1A–C**). Among the latter, classical arborizing vessels are the most distinguishable feature of nodular BCC (**Figure 1A–C**), easily identifiable as larger bright red stem vessels that branch into thinner branches [28]. Arborizing vessels correspond to dilated tumor vessels in the superficial dermis. Although the pigmentation features are the hallmark of pigmented BCC, they may be present in nodular BCC as well.

The most common pigmentation feature of non-sBCC is blue-gray ovoid nests (**Figure 1A** and **C**). Blue-gray ovoid nests are pigmented structures that histopathologically represent pigmented tumor nests invading the dermis. It is worth noting that nBCCs generally appear more pigmented in contrast to sBCCs. In nBCCs, blue-gray pigmentation usually arises in the center of the lesion, whereas maple leaf-like areas, spoke-wheel areas, and concentric structures are closer to the peripheral part of the lesion [30]. Ulcerations are structureless, red to black-red areas in parts of epidermal loss (**Figure 1A**). In some cases, nBCC can even present with shiny white areas and rainbow patterns that occur when the polarized light illuminates vascular structures of the tumor. Further dermatoscopic findings of nBCC include milia-like cysts and multiple aggregated yellow-white globules [31].

Histopathology of nBCC consists of large, round islands of basaloid keratinocytes that extend from the epidermis to the dermis. The nuclei form palisades at the periphery of the lesions, in addition to a lack of central nuclear organization. In some larger tumor islands, necrosis leads to the development of cystic spaces. As a result of ulceration, an adjacent inflammatory infiltrate develops. Additionally, mucin pools may form in cystic or nodulocystic BCCs [32, 33].

In conclusion, the most specific dermatoscopic features of nodular BCC are arborizing vessels together with ulcerations, while some nodular BCCs additionally present with pigmented structures such as blue-gray ovoid nests. The surgery remains the cornerstone of the therapy of nBCC.

3.2 Dermatoscopy of superficial basal cell carcinoma

The superficial basal cell carcinoma clinically presents as well-circumscribed slightly scaly, shiny, red- to pink-colored non-firm macule, patch, or thin plaque (**Figure 2A** and **B**). The diameter of the tumor can range from a few millimeters to several centimeters. Additionally, the pigmented forms of sBCC may have a variable degree of spotty brown to black pigmentation (**Figure 2C** and **D**). Larger sBCC may also exhibit atrophic areas of hypopigmentation [1]. The central part of sBCC often appears atrophic in contrast to the pearly elevated border. The sBCC is locally destructive as it grows gradually and horizontally over time, reaching several centimeters in diameter if not treated. Induration, ulceration, and nodule all rarely appear as a result of the deeper invasion [2].

SBCC is the second most common subtype of BCC developing in approximately 15% of all BCCs. The predilection sites for sBCCs are the trunk and extremities. Often multiple sBCC may occur in one individual [22]. It is important to distinguish sBCC from other BCCs because of the different treatment strategies available for this entity. Currently, depending on the individual clinical presentation, standard surgical excision with postoperative margin evaluation or electrodessication and curettage (EDC) are the treatments of choice for low-risk sBCC, while topical 5-fluorouracil (5-FU) and 5% imiquimod are second-line treatment modalities [23, 34]. The differential diagnosis for sBCC includes actinic keratosis, Bowen's disease, and solitary lichenoid keratosis, in addition to inflammatory diseases such as nummular eczema, psoriasis, and cutaneous lupus erythematosus. Regarding histopathology, sBCC is marked by foci of palisading basaloid cells connecting in a net-like pattern and extending to the papillary dermis [18, 29].

The diagnosis of sBCC is based upon typical clinical features together with dermatoscopic findings and histopathological analysis. Dermatoscopy facilitates the differentiation of sBCC from other BCCs. The main dermatoscopic features of superficial BCC are maple-leaf-like areas, short fine superficial telangiectasias, shiny white-red structureless areas, concentric structures, spoke-wheel

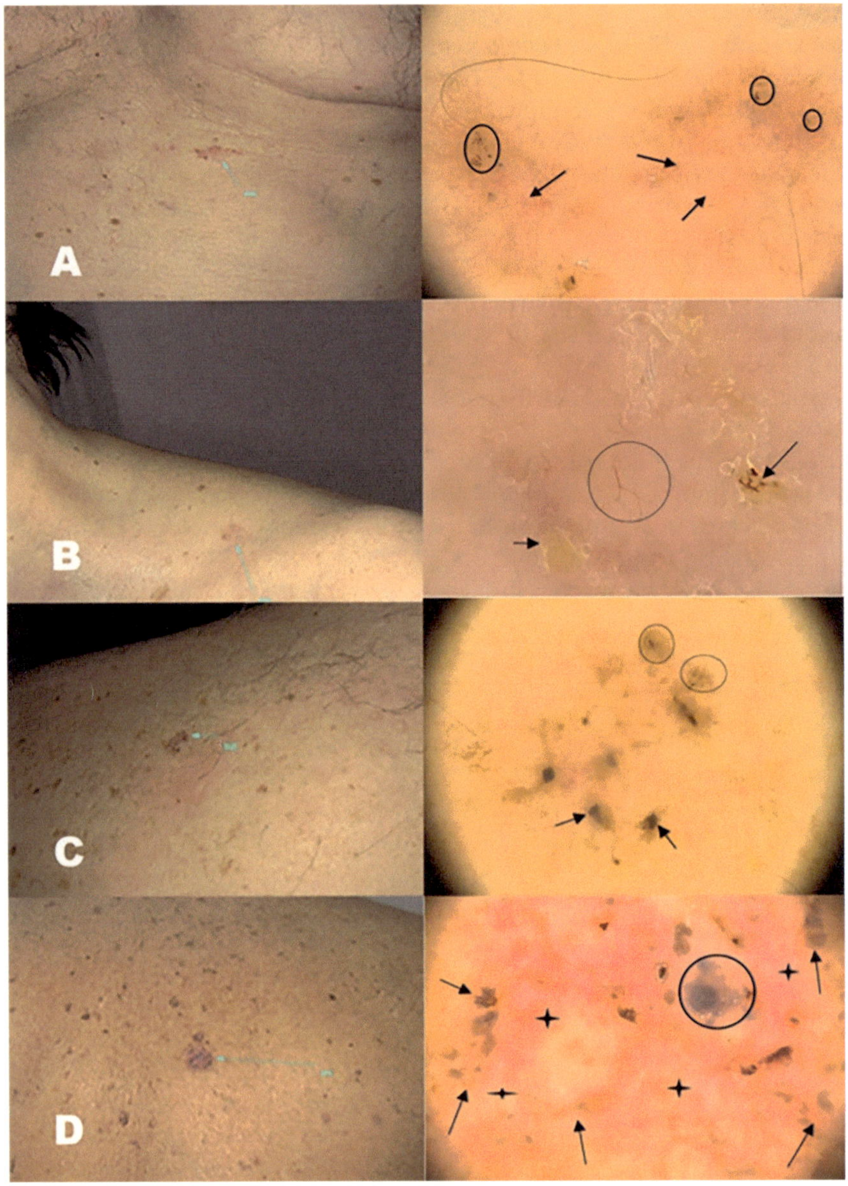

Figure 2.
(A) Left: superficial BCC clinically presented as well-circumscribed red- to pink-colored patch. Right: superficial BCC with short fine telangiectasias (arrows), small brown-gray dots (circles), and white-red structureless areas. (B) Left: well-circumscribed slight scaly, pink-colored macule. Right: arborizing vessels with ramification (black arrows) and multiple yellowish structureless areas representing small ulcerations covered with crust (red arrows). (C) Left: clinical presentation of superficial pigmented BCC. Right: the more experienced dermatoscopist will recognize the leaf-like structures (red circles) and concentric structures (white circles), structures corresponding to dermo-epidermal pigmentation. (D) Left: BCC exhibiting the various amounts of pigment and scale. Right: the dermatoscopic features of superficial BCC are maple leaf-like areas (red circles) and shiny white, red structureless areas (stars) throughout the lesion. In contrast, blue-gray ovoid nests (square) point to the diagnosis of an infiltrative variant of BCC.

areas, and multiple small erosions [29, 35]. However, among the latter, the most positive predictive patterns of sBCC are multiple small erosions and maple leaf-like areas together with short fine superficial telangiectasias (**Figure 2A** and **B**). Under dermatoscopy, short fine telangiectasias appear as fine vascular structures with length up to 1 mm, and only a few branches or commonly, no branching at all [35].

Recently dotted vessels have been described in sBCC located on lower extremities. As the dotted vessels are also a feature of Bowen disease, other features such as white shiny blotches/strands and superficial fine telangiectasia (SFT) should be considered when diagnosing sBCC in this anatomical region [36].

Furthermore, maple-leaf-like areas can be visualized as brown or gray/blue bulbous, leaf-like projections that never arise from the pigmented network or nearby confluent pigmented areas (**Figure 2C** and **D**). Histopathologically, they correspond to pigmented tumor islands that interconnect with lobular extensions. Multiple small erosions are frequently seen in sBCC and they appear as small brown-red to yellow crusts (**Figure 2B**) covering the areas of epidermal loss [30, 37].

Another finding in sBCC is spoke-wheel areas that resemble radial arrays that join at the darker center. They are consistent with tumor nests arising and connecting to the epidermis with finger-like projections and centrally located pigment. The areas of diffuse dermal and tumor fibrosis appear as opaque white to red-colored areas under dermatoscopy, and these are called white-red structureless areas, also familiar as milky-pink areas [38–40]. In addition, short white streaks also correspond to dermal fibrosis and are more commonly seen in sBCCs. Recently, a new dermatoscopic feature of sBCC named negative maple leaf-like areas (NMLLA) has been described. NMLLA are round non-pigmented well-defined bulbous projections similar to maple leaf-like areas on the white-colored background. These areas represent non-pigmented tumor nests at the dermo-epidermal junction and are usually associated with sBCC in the trunk region [41].

Furthermore, loosely arranged, well-defined focused fine brown-to-gray dots can also represent an unspecific feature of sBCC. They correlate with pigment deposition at the dermo-epidermal junction or melanophages in the papillary dermis [42].

Finally, negative predictive patterns of sBCC are ulceration, blue-gray ovoid nests, and arborizing vessels. These findings are suggestive of non-sBCCs subtypes. Among the listed criteria, blue-gray ovoid nests strongly support the diagnosis of infiltrative non-sBCC, which is especially relevant in differentiating clinically flat pigmented lesions. The blue-gray color results from pigment deposition deeper in the dermis, whereas brown pigment corresponds to melanin accumulation at the dermo-epidermal junction [39].

Some authors also suggest clinical subdivision of sBCC to patch, patch-to-plaque, and plaque forms, as more palpable forms of BCC often exhibit dermatoscopic features of nodular BCC (nBCC) [43]. Another helpful finding, highly suggestive of sBCC is multiple small erosions in clinically flat lesions [44].

In brief, pigmented sBCC is defined by patterns corresponding to dermo-epidermal pigmentation, particularly maple leaf-like areas, spoke-wheel, and concentric structures, with the absence of blue-gray ovoid nests, arborizing vessels and ulceration [30]. By adhering to the latter, the diagnosis of sBCC can be made with the sensitivity of 81.9% and specificity of 81.8%. On the contrary, non-pigmented sBCC demonstrates superficial short fine telangiectasia, multiple small erosions, and translucent-to-opaque shiny white-red structureless areas. Dermatoscopy is a reliable method for distinguishing sBCC from other BCCs, and neoplastic and inflammatory disorders. Adding current dermatoscopy algorithms to clinical practice is of crucial importance for making the correct prebiopsy diagnosis [29, 35].

3.3 Dermatoscopy of pigmented BCC

Pigmented BCC is a variant of basal cell carcinoma that histologically exhibits increased melanin pigmentation. It is clinically presented as a nodular pigmented lesion or pigmented macule (**Figure 3A–E**). However, around 30% of BCCs that are clinically classified as non-pigmented reveal pigmented features under dermatoscopy; thus, the pigment-related structures may be found in all BCC subtypes, both superficially and non-superficially [30, 45]. Based

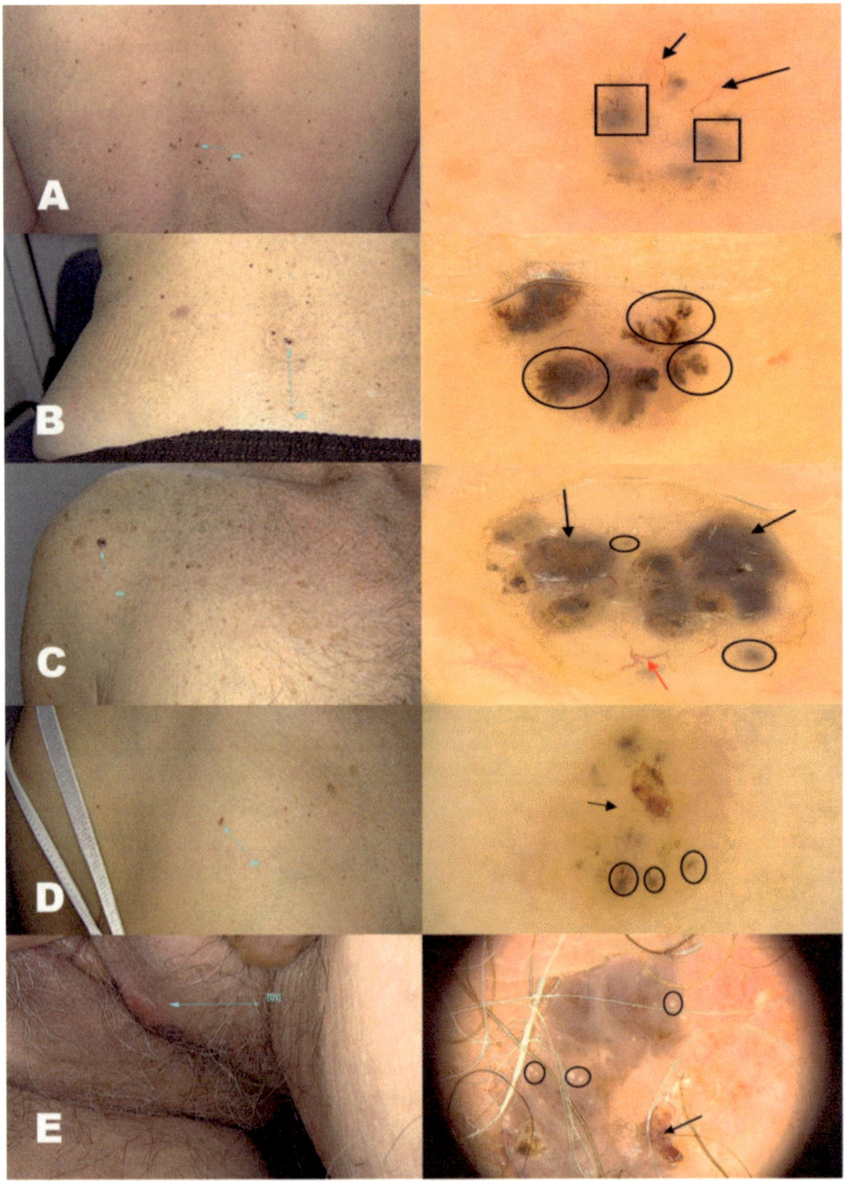

Figure 3.
(A) Left: BCC clinically presented as firm pigmented papule. Right: pigmented basal cell carcinoma with arborizing vessels (arrows) and blue-gray ovoid nests (squares). (B) Left: clinical presentation of pigmented BCC. Right: this pigmented BCC shows the so-called maple leaf-like features (red circles). (C) Left: nodular pigmented BCC clinically presented as firm pigmented papule. Right: the heavily pigmented BCC with large blue-gray blotches (squares), blue-gray ovoid nests, and globules (circle) and arborizing vessels at the periphery of the lesion (arrow). (D) Left: clinical examination revealed small pigmented papule. Right: dermatoscopic picture of classic BCC with spoken wheel structures at the periphery (white circles) and fine arborizing telangiectasia (black arrows) in the middle of the lesion. (E) Left: unusual localization of BCC at labia major. Right: atypical presentation of nodular pigmented BCC with large blue-gray areas, ulceration covered by crust (red arrow), and milia-like cysts (triangles). This nodular BCC is hardly distinguishable from nodular melanoma.

on histopathology correlation, features representing pigment at the dermo-epidermal junction, such as maple-leaf-like areas, spoke-wheel areas, concentric structures, and focus dots, are in brown and appear more frequently in the superficial and infiltrating variant of BCC (**Figure 3B** and **D**). In contrast, features representing pigment in deeper layers of the dermis such as blue-gray ovoid nests and blue-gray globules are in blue or gray, and they are characteristic of the nodular subtype of BCC [37, 39, 45]. Multiple blue-gray globules are defined as numerous, loosely arranged round to oval, well-circumscribed structures similar but smaller than the ovoid nest (**Figure 3A**, **C**, and **E**). They histopathologically correlate with small tumor nests in the papillary or/and reticular dermis. On the other hand, large blue/gray ovoid nests are well-circumscribed, confluent, or near-confluent pigmented or elongated areas, more prominent than globules and not intimately connected to a pigmented tumor body (**Figure 3A**, **C**, and **E**). Regarding pathophysiology, they correspond to large tumor nests with pigment aggregates invading the dermis. Blue-gray blotches together with arborizing vessels represent pathognomonic findings of pigmented basal cell carcinoma. In-focus dot terms describe loosely arranged, well-defined small brown-gray dots, which appear sharply in focus. They correspond to small tumor aggregates in the superficial dermis or at the dermo-epidermal junction, although they may also represent free pigment deposits or melanophages at the junction. Maple leaf-like areas are translucent brown-to-gray/blue peripheral bulbous extensions, mainly localized on the lesion's periphery that never arises from a pigmented network or adjacent confluent pigmented areas (**Figure 3B**). Histologically, they represent pigmented nests at the dermo-epidermal junction and in the superficial papillary dermis. Spoke-wheel areas are well-circumscribed radial projections, usually tan but sometimes blue or gray, meeting at an often darker (dark brown, black, or blue) central axis. They are a rare dermatoscopic feature, highly specific for BCC. Occasionally radial projections are not clearly defined, and they appear as globular structures with a darker center. In such cases, we call them concentric structures [37, 39, 45]. Heavily pigmented BCCs may show dermatoscopic features associated with melanocytic lesions, such as brown globules, a blue-white veil and peppering. It is not always possible to distinguish melanoma from BCC with dermatoscopy; therefore in that clinical setting, the correct management decision is more relevant than the diagnosis (**Figure 3E**).

3.4 Dermatoscopy of infiltrative BCC

Infiltrative BCC is an aggressive and recurrent BCC variant that constitutes 5–10% of the BCCs. It is a histologic variant characterized by invasive growth patterns with clinically indistinct borders. This subtype of BCC is more aggressive and requires wider surgical margins or Mohs surgery, in contrast to non-infiltrative variants such as nodular or superficial BCC, which are commonly treated with standard surgical excision. The most common dermatoscopy features that point to infiltrating growth of BCC are arborizing vessels, fine telangiectasia, shiny white structureless areas, ulceration, and whitish background. Vessels found in the infiltrative variant of BCC are more delicate and more scattered, with fewer branches than nodular subtypes. A pigmented subtype of infiltrative BCC can exhibit blue-gray ovoid nests or multiple blue-gray in-focus dots [28, 37]. The novel dermatoscopic feature linked to the infiltrative form of BCC is called a circumferential stellate pattern. It is defined as a geometric star-shaped pattern extending outward from the circumferential peripheral edge of the tumor and identified by white lines, vessels, or uneven skin surface morphology [46].

3.5 Dermatoscopy of morpheaform/sclerodermiform BCC

Morpheaform BCC is an uncommon variant of BCC in which tumor cells induce proliferation of fibroblasts within the dermis and an increased collagen deposition with sclerosis that clinically resembles a scar. The histologic extent often exceeds the clinical impression, leading to high recurrence rates after standard excision. Morheaform BCC displays dermatoscopic features at a later stage of development than other subtypes of BCCs [47]. Approximately 75% of tumors show a structureless hypopigmented porcelain area. Arborizing vessels are expected in morpheaform BCC, and they tend to have less evident branching. This subtype of BCC is rarely pigmented, but when they are, dermoscopy shows blue-gray ovoid nests [36]. If pink-white areas and fine arborizing vessels are seen in high-risk zones such as the nose, cheek, and periauricular area, clinician should consider a diagnosis of sclerodermiforme BCC.

3.6 Dermatoscopy of fibroepithelial BCC

Another uncommon variant of BCC is fibroepithelial BCC. Fibroepithelial BCC, also known as Pinkus tumor, clinically appears as erythematous, flesh-colored dome-shaped papule or plaque. Differential diagnoses include benign skin lesions such as dermal nevus, fibroma, seborrheic keratosis, and even malignant tumors such as amelanotic melanoma [48]. Dermatoscopy patterns seen in fibroepithelioma of Pinkus are fine arborizing vessels that have less evident ramification and are smaller in caliber in contrast to telangiectasia seen in other forms of BCC accompanied by white streaks under polarized dermatoscopy that are called crystalline structures similar to those in other forms of BCC. Pigmented variants show brown-gray structureless areas and blue-gray dots. Other common but unspecific findings are milia-like cysts and ulceration [48, 49].

3.7 Dermatoscopy of basosquamous carcinoma

Basosquamous carcinoma (BsC) is a controversial entity and has both diagnostic and therapeutic challenges. BsC combines histopathologic and dermoscopic characteristics of basal cell carcinoma (BCC) and squamous cell carcinoma (SCC) [1]. Like SCC, BsC is more locally invasive and aggressive, and metastasizes more often than other forms of BCC. Dermatoscopy features comprise both features of BCC and SCC. Therefore, besides arborizing vessels, ulceration, and blood crust that are standard features of BCC, BsC is characterized by keratin masses, surface scaling, and white structureless areas, and dermoscopic features are mainly seen in SCC [27].

3.8 The dermatoscopic findings of other uncommon variants of BCC

The nevoid BCC that typically develops in Gorlin-Goltz patients together with palmar pits may show blue-gray dots, globules, or nests and arborizing vessels at the periphery.

Micronodular basal cell carcinoma is a histopathological term that applies to BCCs in which smaller aggregations of basaloid cells infiltrate the dermis. They have destructive behavior, with subclinical spread and high rates of recurrence. Only a few studies have specifically analyzed dermatoscopic features of micronodular BCCs. The main features were truncated vessels and multiple blue-gray globules [42].

BCCs with a linear appearance are sporadic, sometimes seen in association with different histological subtypes. The most frequently affected sites are the periorbital area and the neck. The linear subtype of BCC may show any dermatoscopic features associated with BCC in general.

4. Conclusion

Generally observing, classic arborizing vessels are typically found in a nodular variant of BCC, while short fine telangiectasia points forward the superficial form of BCC. Structures associated with pigment could be roughly divided into two categories based on melanin deposition. All dermatoscopic subtypes of BCC can exhibit various amounts of pigment. Maple leaf-like areas, spoke-wheel areas, concentric structures, and in-focus dots indicate the presence of melanin at the dermo-epidermal junction and are a feature of superficial BCC. On the other hand, large blue-gray ovoid nests and multiple blue-gray dots and globules correspond to melanin at the dermal level. They are the characteristic of a non-superficial variant of BCC. Spoke-wheel areas are a rare dermatoscopic feature, but they are highly particular for BCC. Ulceration represents a loss of epidermis and portion of the dermis and is primarily seen in nodular lesions. Ulcerated areas are frequently covered with coagulated blood or crust, sometimes making it difficult for further dermatoscopic review. Multiple small erosions are the characteristic of a superficial variant of BCC, and they are smaller than ulcerations and clinically observed as a yellowish crust.

Diagnosis of BCC is not established on a single dermatoscopy feature, but rather on the coexistence of several dermatoscopic features together with clinical presentation. Histopathology essentially yields the final and decisive diagnosis. Besides a prominent position in diagnosis, dermatoscopy holds an essential role in managing BCC, significantly improving the treatment and post-treatment outcome assessment, possessing a beneficial role during all the stages of BCC management.

Author details

Tina Zagar[1], Nika Hlaca[1,2]* and Larisa Prpic-Massari[1,2]

1 Department of Dermatovenerology, Clinical Hospital Centre Rijeka, Rijeka, Croatia

2 Medical Faculty, University of Rijeka, Rijeka, Croatia

*Address all correspondence to: nika.hlaca@uniri.hr

References

[1] Tan ST, Ghaznawie M, Heenan PJ, Dosan R. Basal cell carcinoma arises from interfollicular layer of epidermis. Journal of Oncology. 2018;**26**:3098940. DOI: 10.1155/2018/3098940

[2] Scrivener Y, Grosshans E, Cribier B. Variations of basal cell carcinomas according to gender, age, location and histopathological subtype. The British Journal of Dermatology. 2002;**147**:41-47. DOI: 10.1046/j.1365-2133.2002.04804.x

[3] Verkouteren JAC, Ramdas KHR, Wakkee M, Nijsten T. Epidemiology of basal cell carcinoma: Scholarly review. The British Journal of Dermatology. 2017;**177**:359

[4] Reinau D, Surber C, Jick SS, Meier CR. Epidemiology of basal cell carcinoma in the United Kingdom: Incidence, lifestyle factors, and comorbidities. British Journal of Cancer. 2014;**111**:203

[5] Savoye I, Olsen CM, Whiteman DC, et al. Patterns of ultraviolet radiation exposure and skin cancer risk: The E3N-SunExp study. Journal of Epidemiology. 2018;**28**:27

[6] Gandini S, Doré JF, Autier P, et al. Epidemiological evidence of carcinogenicity of sunbed use and of efficacy of preventive measures. Journal of the European Academy of Dermatology and Venereology. 2019;**33**(Suppl 2):57

[7] Robinson SN, Zens MS, Perry AE, et al. Photosensitizing agents and the risk of non-melanoma skin cancer: A population-based case-control study. The Journal of Investigative Dermatology. 2013;**133**:1950

[8] Watt TC, Inskip PD, Stratton K, et al. Radiation-related risk of basal cell carcinoma: A report from the Childhood Cancer Survivor Study. Journal of the National Cancer Institute. 2012;**104**:1240

[9] Silverberg MJ, Leyden W, Warton EM, et al. HIV infection status, immunodeficiency, and the incidence of non-melanoma skin cancer. Journal of the National Cancer Institute. 2013;**105**:350

[10] Castori M, Morrone A, Kanitakis J, Grammatico P. Genetic skin diseases predisposing to basal cell carcinoma. European Journal of Dermatology. 2012;**22**:299

[11] MacDonald DS. A systematic review of the literature of nevoid basal cell carcinoma syndrome affecting East Asians and North Europeans. Oral Surgery, Oral Medicine, Oral Pathology, Oral Radiology. 2015;**120**:396

[12] Berlin NL, Cartmel B, Leffell DJ, et al. Family history of skin cancer is associated with early-onset basal cell carcinoma independent of MC1R genotype. Cancer Epidemiology. 2015;**39**:1078

[13] Pellegrini C, Maturo MG, Di Nardo L, et al. Understanding the molecular genetics of basal cell carcinoma. International Journal of Molecular Sciences. 2017;**18**:2485

[14] Epstein EH. Basal cell carcinomas: Attack of the hedgehog. Nature Reviews. Cancer. 2008;**8**:743

[15] Stacey SN, Sulem P, Jonasdottir A, et al. A germline variant in the TP53 polyadenylation signal confers cancer susceptibility. Nature Genetics. 2011;**43**:1098

[16] Lin Y, Chahal HS, Wu W, et al. Association study of genetic variation in DNA repair pathway genes and risk of basal cell carcinoma. International Journal of Cancer. 2017;**141**:952

[17] Bonilla X, Parmentier L, King B, et al. Genomic analysis identifies new drivers and progression pathways in skin basal cell carcinoma. Nature Genetics. 2016;**48**:398

[18] Cameron MC, Lee E, Hibler BP, et al. Basal cell carcinoma: Epidemiology; pathophysiology; clinical and histological subtypes; and disease associations. Journal of the American Academy of Dermatology. 2019;**80**:303-317. DOI: 10.1016/j.jaad.2018.03.060

[19] Wang YJ, Tang TY, Wang JY, et al. Genital basal cell carcinoma, a different pathogenesis from sun-exposed basal cell carcinoma? A case-control study of 30 cases. Journal of Cutaneous Pathology. 2018;**45**:688-695

[20] Reiter O, Mimouni I, Gdalevich M, et al. The diagnostic accuracy of dermoscopy for basal cell carcinoma: A systematic review and meta-analysis. Journal of the American Academy of Dermatology. 2019;**80**:1380

[21] Haws AL, Rojano R, Tahan SR, Phung TL. Accuracy of biopsy sampling for subtyping basal cell carcinoma. Journal of the American Academy of Dermatology. 2012;**66**:106

[22] Bastiaens MT, Hoefnagel JJ, Bruijn JA, et al. Differences in age, site distribution, and sex between nodular and superficial basal cell carcinoma indicate different types of tumors. The Journal of Investigative Dermatology. 1998;**110**:880-884

[23] The NCCN Basal Cell Skin Cancer Clinical Practice Guidelines in Oncology (Version 2.2021 – February 25, 2021). © 2021 National Comprehensive Cancer Network, Inc. Available from: http://www.nccn.org

[24] Urech M, Kyrgidis A, Argenziano G, et al. Dermoscopic ulceration is a predictor of basal cell carcinoma response to imiquimod: A retrospective study. Acta Dermato-Venereologica. 2017;**97**:117-119. DOI: 10.2340/00015555-2464

[25] Christensen E, Warloe T, Kroon S, et al. Guidelines for practical use of MAL-PDT in non-melanoma skin cancer. Journal of the European Academy of Dermatology and Venereology. 2010;**24**:505-512. DOI: 10.1111/j.1468-3083.2009.03430.x

[26] Apalla Z, Lallas A, Tzellos T, et al. Applicability of dermoscopy for evaluation of patients' response to nonablative therapies for the treatment of superficial basal cell carcinoma. The British Journal of Dermatology. 2014;**170**:809-815. DOI: 10.1111/bjd.12749

[27] Costantino D, Lowe L, Brown DL. Basosquamous carcinoma—An under-recognized, high-risk cutaneous neoplasm: Case study and review of the literature. Journal of Plastic, Reconstructive & Aesthetic Surgery. 2006;**59**:424-428

[28] Zalaudek I, Kreusch J, Giacomel J, et al. How to diagnose nonpigmented skin tumors: A review of vascular structures seen with dermoscopy: Part II. Nonmelanocytic skin tumors. Journal of the American Academy of Dermatology. 2010;**63**:377-386; quiz 87-8

[29] Pan Y, Chamberlain AJ, Bailey M, et al. Dermatoscopy aids in the diagnosis of the solitary red scaly patch or plaque-features distinguishing superficial basal cell carcinoma, intraepidermal carcinoma, and psoriasis. Journal of the American Academy of Dermatology. 2008;**59**:268-274

[30] Lallas A, Tzellos T, Kyrgidis A, et al. Accuracy of dermoscopic criteria for discriminating superficial from other subtypes of basal cell carcinoma. Journal of the American Academy of Dermatology. 2014;**70**:303-311

[31] Bellucci C, Arginelli F, Bassoli S, Magnoni C, Seidenari S. Dermoscopic yellow structures in basal cell carcinoma. Journal of the European Academy of Dermatology and Venereology. 2014;**28**:651-654. DOI: 10.1111/jdv.12092

[32] Lallas A, Argenziano G, Zendri E, et al. Update on non-melanoma skin cancer and the value of dermoscopy in its diagnosis and treatment monitoring. Expert Review of Anticancer Therapy. 2013;**13**:541-558

[33] Lallas A, Moscarella E, Argenziano G, et al. Dermoscopy of uncommon skin tumours. The Australasian Journal of Dermatology. 2014;**55**:53-62. DOI: 10.1111/ajd.12074

[34] Williams HC, Bath-Hextall F, Ozolins M, et al. Surgery versus 5% imiquimod for nodular and superficial basal cell carcinoma: 5-year results of the SINS randomized controlled trial. The Journal of Investigative Dermatology. 2017;**137**:614-619

[35] Altamura D, Menzies SW, Argenziano G, et al. Dermatoscopy of basal cell carcinoma: Morphologic variability of global and local features and accuracy of diagnosis. Journal of the American Academy of Dermatology. 2010;**62**:67-75

[36] Papageorgiou C, Apalla Z, Variaah G, et al. Accuracy of dermoscopic criteria for the differentiation between superficial basal cell carcinoma and Bowen's disease. Journal of the European Academy of Dermatology and Venereology. 2018;**32**:1914-1919

[37] Lallas A, Apalla Z, Argenziano G, et al. The dermatoscopic universe of basal cell carcinoma. Dermatology Practical & Conceptual. 2014;**4**:11-24

[38] Marghoob AA, Malvehy J, Braun RP. An Atlas of Dermoscopy. 2nd ed. Oxford: CRC Press; 2012

[39] Demirtasoglu M, Ilknur T, Lebe B, et al. Evaluation of dermoscopic and histopathologic features and their correlations in pigmented basal cell carcinomas. Journal of the European Academy of Dermatology and Venereology. 2006;**20**:916-920

[40] Peris K, Altobelli E, Ferrari A, et al. Interobserver agreement on dermoscopic features of pigmented basal cell carcinoma. Dermatologic Surgery. 2002;**28**:643-645

[41] Imbernón-Moya A, Sidro M, Malvehy J, Puig S. Negative maple-leaf-like areas: A new clue for basal cell carcinoma margin recognition. The British Journal of Dermatology. 2016;**175**:818-820. DOI: 10.1111/bjd.14620

[42] Lallas A, Apalla Z, Ioannides D, et al. Dermoscopy in the diagnosis and management of basal cell carcinoma. Future Oncology. 2015;**11**:2975-2984

[43] Scalvenzi M, Lembo S, Francia MG, et al. Dermoscopic patterns of superficial basal cell carcinoma. International Journal of Dermatology. 2008;**47**:1015-1018

[44] Ahnlide I, Zalaudek I, Nilsson F, et al. Preoperative prediction of histopathological outcome in basal cell carcinoma: Flat surface and multiple small erosions predict superficial basal cell carcinoma in lighter skin types. The British Journal of Dermatology. 2016;**175**:751-761. DOI: 10.1111/bjd.14499

[45] Lallas A, Argenziano G, Kyrgidis A, et al. Dermoscopy uncovers clinically undetectable pigmentation in basal cell carcinoma. The British Journal of Dermatology. 2014;**170**:192-195

[46] Pyne JH, Fishburn P, Dicker A, et al. Infiltrating Basal cell carcinoma: A stellate peri-tumor dermatoscopy pattern as a clue to diagnosis.

Dermatology Practical & Conceptual. 2015;**5**:21-26

[47] Husein-ElAhmed H. Sclerodermiform basal cell carcinoma: How much can we rely on dermatoscopy to differentiate from non-aggressive basal cell carcinoma? Analysis of 1256 cases. Anais Brasileiros de Dermatologia. 2018;**93**:229-232

[48] Viera M, Amini S, Huo R, et al. A new look at fibroepithelioma of pinkus: Features on confocal microscopy. The Journal of Clinical and Aesthetic Dermatology. 2008;**1**:42-44

[49] Zalaudek I, Leinweber B, Ferrara G, et al. Dermoscopy of fibroepithelioma of pinkus. Journal of the American Academy of Dermatology. 2005;**52**: 168-169

Chapter 3

Dermatoscopy of Facial Non-Pigmented Actinic Keratosis and Intraepidermal Carcinoma

Alise Balcere

Abstract

Dermatoscopy improves the diagnostic accuracy of non-pigmented facial lesions, including actinic keratosis (AK) and intraepidermal carcinoma (IEC) and helps to differentiate them from common invasive malignancies such as basal cell carcinoma and invasive squamous cell carcinoma. The most common dermatoscopic features characterizing AK are background erythema/erythematous pseudonetwork, white follicular openings/targetoid hair follicles, surface scales, rosettes, fine, linear, wavy vessels, microerosions and sun-damaged surrounding skin. In comparison, the most common dermatoscopic features of IEC are background erythema, red starburst pattern, surface scale, dotted/glomerular vessels, hairpin vessels, microerosions/ulcerations and targetoid hair follicles. The practice of recognizing these features in dermatoscopic images is a useful tool in the armamentarium of a clinician examining skin lesions.

Keywords: actinic keratosis, erythematous facial lesions, squamous cell carcinoma in situ, bowenoid actinic keratosis

1. Introduction

Actinic keratosis (AK) and other forms of squamous cell carcinoma (SCC) in situ are among the most common lesions in dermatological practice and are primarily the result of cumulative UV damage. The clinical relevance of accurate diagnosis relies on several factors. Firstly, misdiagnosing an inflammatory disease as an AK would lead to unnecessary and possibly harmful usage of destructive therapies on benign lesions. Secondly, AK is commonly a lesion in a field of sun-damaged skin, and among other lesions associated with chronic sun damage, some small clinically indistinguishable carcinomas may rest. Moreover, AK, although a common lesion, might progress to invasive SCC with gradual changes that can be visualized under a dermatoscope [1]. Furthermore, studies have shown that most SCCs arise from or in close proximity to AK and that dermatoscopy aids in differentiation between AK and SCC [2, 3]. Therefore, dermatoscopy is a useful tool for a clinician examining non-pigmented facial lesions allowing to differentiate between them.

Several forms of in situ SCC that are united by atypical keratinocytes in the epidermis but vary clinically, dermatoscopically, and histopathologically have been recognized [4]. Actinic keratosis (AK) and intraepidermal carcinoma (IEC) are the two main types of SCC in situ affecting facial skin. Much less common forms include arsenical keratosis, radiation keratosis (caused by ionizing radiation), and hydrocarbon keratosis, in which dermatoscopic differences have not been described [5]. The following chapter will provide an overview of the clinical and dermatoscopic features that characterize different forms of AK and IEC of the face, including the dermatoscopic progression model from AK to invasive SCC.

2. Definition of actinic keratosis and intraepidermal carcinoma

The differentiation between AK and IEC relies on their histopathologic characteristics.

AK is also called solar or senile keratosis, SCC in situ AK-type, or keratinocytic intraepidermal neoplasia and represents a common lesion on chronically sun-damaged skin of fair skinned individuals. Histopathologically, AK presents as atypia of basal keratinocytes with loss of polarization, crowding, and overlapping that can extend up to near full thickness atypia in advanced lesions [5–8].

IEC is an intraepithelial SCC exhibiting full-thickness cellular dysplasia [9]. However, other synonyms employed for extragenital full-thickness intraepidermal carcinoma are Bowen's disease, in situ SCC, cutaneous SCC in situ, and intraepithelial SCC [1]. It is noteworthy that in comparison with other types of SCC in situ, Bowen's disease has been defined as SCC in situ arising on sun-protected skin, without field damage and possibly without association with HPV, although previously suggested otherwise [10–12]. For the consistency of this chapter, the term "*intraepidermal carcinoma*" will be used to describe facial intraepithelial SCC exhibiting full-thickness cellular dysplasia.

3. Diagnosing AK and IEC

Actinic keratosis in the majority of cases can be diagnosed clinically. Nevertheless, the clinical description of an erythematous macule or patch with a superficial scale may correspond to many other skin lesions and dermatoses. Studies [13, 14] examining the diagnostic precision of clinically diagnosed AK have reported misdiagnosis rates of approximately 10%. The main biopsy diagnoses in cases of misdiagnosis were SCC in situ, SCC with superficial invasion, seborrheic keratosis, basal cell carcinoma, and other benign skin lesions and dermatoses such as subacute spongiotic dermatitis, rosacea, solar elastosis, scars and verrucae plana. Pivotal differential diagnosis of AK is invasive SCC that can mimic AK if presenting as an erythematous macule. It has been shown that 1.5% of clinically diagnosed AK lesions identified by board-certified dermatologist were SCCs with superficial invasion on histologic assessment [13]. In comparison, dermatoscopy improves the diagnostic accuracy of both AK and SCC. A recent systematic review and study by Huerta-Brogeras *et al*. showed sensitivity up to 98.7% and specificity up to 95% if AK is diagnosed with dermatoscopy [15, 16].

Diagnosis of IEC is based on clinical, dermatoscopic, and histopathologic features.

3.1 Clinical features of AK and IEC

The most frequent presentation of both AK and IEC is a variably erythematous scaly patch or slightly elevated plaque [17]. AK is either single or multiple, while IEC is usually a single lesion. In comparison with AK, IEC is often an indurated lesion on palpation. Both lesions are asymptomatic in most of the cases, although some patients experience discomfort, such as burning, pain, bleeding, and pruritus [6]. It has been noted that pain can be equally present in both AK and IEC, but is more common in invasive SCC [18].

A broad and useful tool for clinical description of the thickness of AK is a classification by Olsen *et al.* [19]. In this classification:

- Grade 1 AKs are mild - slightly palpable, better felt than seen.
- Grade 2 AKs are moderately thick that are easily seen and felt.
- Grade 3 AKs are severe - very thick, hyperkeratotic, and obvious AK.

However, this clinical classification cannot reliably predict the histological grade proposed by Roewert-Huber *et al.* that could justify the classical progression model of AK to invasive SCC through clinical thickening and histopathological upward extension of atypical keratinocytes before invasion. It has been shown that only 26% of Olsen grade 1 lesions were grade 1 on histopathology with atypical keratinocytes in the basal and suprabasal layers of the epidermis, 75% of Olsen grade 2 lesions were grade II on histopathology with atypical keratinocytes extending to the lower two-thirds of the epidermis and only 14% of Olsen grade 3 lesions had corresponding grade III on histopathology with atypical keratinocytes extending to more than two thirds of the full thickness of the epidermis [8, 20].

3.2 Dermatoscopic features of AK and IEC

For the description of dermatoscopic features of AK and IEC, both metaphoric and descriptive language can be used. Definitions of the main metaphoric and descriptive terms are given in **Table 1**.

Main dermatoscopic features of AK are depicted in **Table 2**. Main dermatoscopic features of IEC are depicted in **Table 3**.

Metaphoric/descriptive terms	Definition
Red pseudonetwork	Marked pink-to-red background erythema surrounding accentuated hair follicles
Red starburst pattern	Radially arranged structureless red lines or hairpin vessels that surround a yellow to white structureless scaly center and that resemble an overall starburst appearance
Rosettes	Four bright white dots or clods arranged together as a square (or 4-leaf clover)
Shiny white streaks	Short discrete white lines oriented parallel and orthogonal (perpendicular) to each other seen only under polarized dermatoscopy
Strawberry pattern	Red pseudonetwork in combination with targetoid hair follicles
Targetoid hair follicle	Yellowish keratotic plug within a prominent hair follicle opening surrounded by a white halo
White circles	Bright white circles surrounding an orange/yellow keratin plug

Table 1.
Standardized terms of common dermatoscopic features for AK and IEC [18, 21–23].

Classic AK	**Most common dermatoscopic findings**	
	• Background erythema/erythematous pseudonetwork	**Strawberry pattern**
	• Follicular openings/ targetoid hair follicles	
	• Surface scales ○ Yellow-white opaque scales ○ Diffuse/discrete scales • Rosettes • Fine, linear, wavy vessels • Microerosions • Sun damaged surrounding skin	
	Less common, but possible findings	**Structure is more characteristic to**
	• Central scale	IEC, SCC, KA
	• Dotted/glomerular vessels	IEC
	• White structureless areas (common in Korean patients)	SCC, KA
	A rare finding	**Structure is more characteristic to**
	• Central ulceration	SCC, KA
	• Linear-irregular vessels	KA, SCC
	• Hairpin vessels	SCC, KA, IEC
	• Red starburst pattern	IEC, SCC
	• Shiny white streaks	Dermatofibroma, scar, BCC
Bowenoid AK	**Most common dermatoscopic findings**	
	• Glomerular vessels regularly distributed	
	• Surface scale	
Hyperkeratotic AK	**Most common dermatoscopic findings**	
	• Marked hyperkeratosis seen as white-yellow structureless areas preventing visualization of underlying structures	

Table 2.
Dermatoscopic features of AK categorized in three groups according to their prevalence. The most common dermatoscopic findings – Features present in almost all to the majority of AKs. Less common, but possible findings – Present in some AKs, although more common and characteristic for other lesions. A rare finding – Sometimes present in AK, but a differential diagnosis is much more likely. Abbreviations: AK – Actinic keratosis; IEC – Intraepidermal carcinoma; KA - Keratoacanthoma; SCC – Squamous cell carcinoma; BCC – Basal cell carcinoma [1, 6, 15, 22–26].

3.2.1 Characteristics of specific features

3.2.1.1 Erythematous pseudonetwork

Erythematous pseudonetwork can be defined as a marked pink-to-red background erythema formed by fine wavy telangiectatic vessels surrounding accentuated hair follicles [23]. It is one of the most common and characteristic findings of AK.

IEC	Most common dermatoscopic findings	

	• Background erythema
	• Red starburst pattern
	• Surface scales
	  ○ Yellow-white opaque scales
	  ○ Central scale
	  ○ Diffuse/discrete scales
	• Dotted/glomerular vessels
	• Hairpin vessels
	• Microerosions/ulcerations
	• Targetoid hair follicles	

	Less common, but possible findings	**Structure is more characteristic to**
	• Rosettes	
	• Central keratin mass	KA, SCC
	• Red pseudonetwork	AK
	A rare finding	**Structure is more characteristic to**
	• White structureless areas	KA, SCC
	• Linear-irregular vessels	KA, SCC
	• Central ulceration	BCC, SCC, KA

Table 3.
Dermatoscopic features of IEC categorized in three groups according to their prevalence. The most common dermatoscopic findings – Features present in almost all to majority of IECs. Less common, but possible findings – Present in some IECs, although more common and characteristic for other lesions. A rare finding – Sometimes present in IEC, but a differential diagnosis is much more likely. Abbreviations: AK – Actinic keratosis; IEC – Intraepidermal carcinoma; KA - Keratoacanthoma; SCC – Squamous cell carcinoma; BCC – Basal cell carcinoma [1].

3.2.1.2 Targetoid hair follicles

Targetoid hair follicles are formed by yellowish keratotic plugs within the hair follicles and surrounded by a whitish halo. This feature is particularly common for AK on the nose and hyperkeratotic AK [23].

3.2.1.3 Strawberry pattern

Strawberry pattern (**Figure 1**) is a composite appearance of reddish pseudonetwork and hair follicles. This pattern is present in up to 95% of AK [23].

3.2.1.4 Surface scales

Scales are one of the most common features of AK and correlate with hyperkeratosis and parakeratosis on histopathology [21]. The distribution is usually diffuse throughout the lesion, although some lesions can be partly scaly (**Figure 1**) and a central scale is common for hyperkeratotic lesions. The color of the scales varies from white to yellow and an accumulation of exogenous pigment has been reported [27].

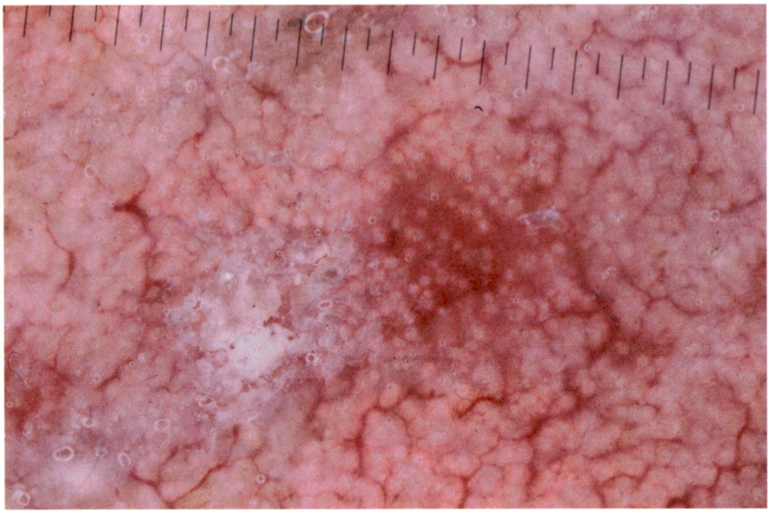

Figure 1.
Dermatoscopic image of an AK. White scales limiting visualization of the underlying structures are seen on the left side of the picture, while a typical strawberry pattern with erythematous pseudonetwork and targetoid hair follicles are seen on the right side.

3.2.1.5 Rosettes

Rosettes are also named 4-dotted-clods in descriptive terminology. Rosettes are a clue for keratinizing neoplasms, although they can also be observed in several other conditions including basal cell carcinoma, melanoma, melanocytic nevus, dermatofibroma, scar, molluscum contagiosum, actinically damaged skin and cicatricial alopecia of lichen planopilaris [28]. The dermatopathological correlate of 4-dotted-clods in AK is horizontally arranged alternating hyperkeratotic and parakeratotic corneal layers in the follicular infundibula associated with mild peri-follicular fibrosis [28]. It has also been proposed that smaller 4-dotted-clods are caused by the concentric horn in the follicle at the infundibular level, whereas larger ones are caused by concentric fibrosis around the follicle [29].

3.2.1.6 Fine, linear, wavy vessels

Focused linear wavy vessels surrounding the hair follicles was found in more than 80% of facial AKs in a study by Zalaudek *et al*. These peculiar linear, wavy vessels of facial AK clearly differ in morphology from the arborizing vessels of vessels of nodular basal, short fine telangiectatic vessels of superficial basal cell carcinoma, and regular hairpin vessels that are characteristic of seborrhoeic keratosis. Furthermore, wavy vessels typically encircle the hair follicles as single and uniform units, which contrasts with the irregularly sized and distributed linear irregular vessels that can be seen in amelanotic/hypomelanotic melanoma, areas of regression in melanoma, or invasive SCC [23].

3.2.1.7 Microerosions

Microerosions are small erosions on the surface of the lesion seen under a dermatoscope. Microerosions are twice as common in IEC in comparison with AK, but are also a common feature of superficial basal cell carcinoma [1].

3.2.1.8 Shiny white streaks

Shiny white streaks (SWS) are also known as chrysalis or crystalline structures by their metaphoric terms. Dermatoscopically, SWS are only visible in a polarized light dermatoscopy as white, perpendicular, few millimeters long lines. Histopathologically, SWS are caused by polarization of thickened hyaline fibrous bundles and therefore considered as a dermatoscopic sign of dermal fibrosis. Shiny white streaks have been reported in a variety of skin lesions, mainly dermatofibromas, scars, basal cell carcinomas, lichen planus like keratosis, invasive melanoma, melanoma metastasis and sometimes even solar lentigo and intradermal nevus. In addition, it has been reported that SWS might be less common in inflamed lesions [22, 25, 29–31].

3.2.1.9 Sun damaged surrounding skin

The importance of recognizing the features of the surrounding skin is based on several factors. First of all, AK quite commonly has a confluent solar lentigo on the border. Secondly, it has been hypothesized that humans focus on the lesion and not on the surrounding skin and therefore are outperformed by artificial intelligence in the precision of AK diagnosis. Moreover, teaching medical students to pay attention to chronic sun damage in the background improved the frequency of correct diagnoses of pigmented actinic keratoses from 32.5% to 47.3% [26]. In addition, lesions arising in field cancerization have a higher potential for malignant progression. The latter has been recognized in a new nomenclature of keratinocyte cancers by Conforti *et al.* According to the authors, all keratinocyte cancers should be classified in two groups - 'cSCC+field' for keratinocyte cancers arising in the presence of AK within the field of cancerization and 'cSCC-field' for keratinocyte cancers arising in the absence of AK or field cancerization [32].

3.2.1.10 Red starburst pattern

Red starburst pattern can be defined as radially arranged structureless red lines or hairpin vessels that surround a yellow to white structureless scaly center and that resemble an overall starburst appearance (**Figure 2**). Red starburst pattern is equally common in IEC and invasive SCC, and less common in AK [1].

3.2.1.11 Dotted/glomerular vessels

Dotted vessels are tiny red dots densely aligned next to each other [1]. Glomerular vessels are larger-caliber reddish dots formed by tortuous capillaries curled up into a ball and resembling the glomerular apparatus of the kidneys. Glomerular vessels are specific for Bowen's disease, if located in clusters and bowenoid AK, if distributed regularly. Glomerular vessels can also be present in stasis dermatitis, psoriasis, irritated seborrheic keratosis, superficial basal cell carcinoma and melanoma [33–35]. The combination of clustered dotted/glomerular vessels and hyperkeratosis has been previously shown to achieve a 98% diagnostic probability for IEC [1, 35].

3.2.1.12 Hairpin vessels

Hairpin vessels are vessels that double back on themselves and are seen as loops when they are oblique to the surface of the lesion. Hairpin vessels are a common feature of keratinizing tumors and are a hallmark of seborrheic keratosis in which

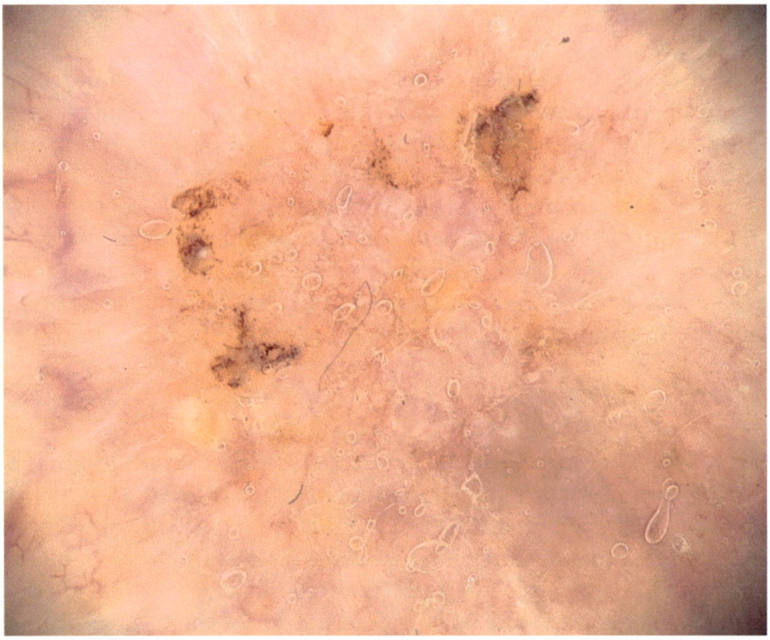

Figure 2.
Dermatoscopic image of IEC presenting with red starburst appearance formed by red and white radially arranged lines and central pink structureless clods, yellow scales, and hemorrhagic crusts.

they are usually regularly distributed and surrounded by a white halo. Hairpin vessels are a rare but possible finding in AK and a common finding in IEC and SCC. Hairpin vessels are associated with progression of IEC to invasive SCC and clinically thicker lesions. Positive predictive value of hairpin vessels for seborrheic keratosis is 70%, contrasting with only 13.3% for squamous cell carcinoma [1, 33].

3.2.2 Variants of AK

Apart from classical AK, other forms categorized histopathologically are hypertrophic, atrophic, bowenoid, acantholytic, pigmented, lichenoid, and proliferative variants, although in this grading system overlap of histologic subtypes may occur in a single lesion [36].

Atrophic AK. In this form, the lesion has an atrophic epidermis on histopathology [5]. According to one study, atrophic type AK more commonly presents with red pseudonetwork [37].

Bowenoid AK has a characteristic dermatoscopic feature of glomerular vessels regularly distributed along the lesion (**Figures 3** and **4**), thus differentiating it from Bowen's disease, whose vessels are irregularly distributed and grouped [6].

Hyperkeratotic AK presents with a nonspecific dermatoscopic pattern due to hyperkeratosis, which prevents visualization of the underlying structures [6]. In addition, it has been shown that the surface keratin of AK can accumulate exogenous pigmentation, particularly from broad spectrum sunscreens containing titanium dioxide. Such a specific feature of bright arctic-blue or greenish-blue color of AK on polarized light dermatoscopy has been described and named an "iceberg sign" [27].

Lichenoid AK clinically presents with pronounced erythema around the base of the lesion secondary to an underlying lichenoid infiltrate on histopathology [5]. Dermatoscopically, lichenoid AK might also present with a more intense erythematous background.

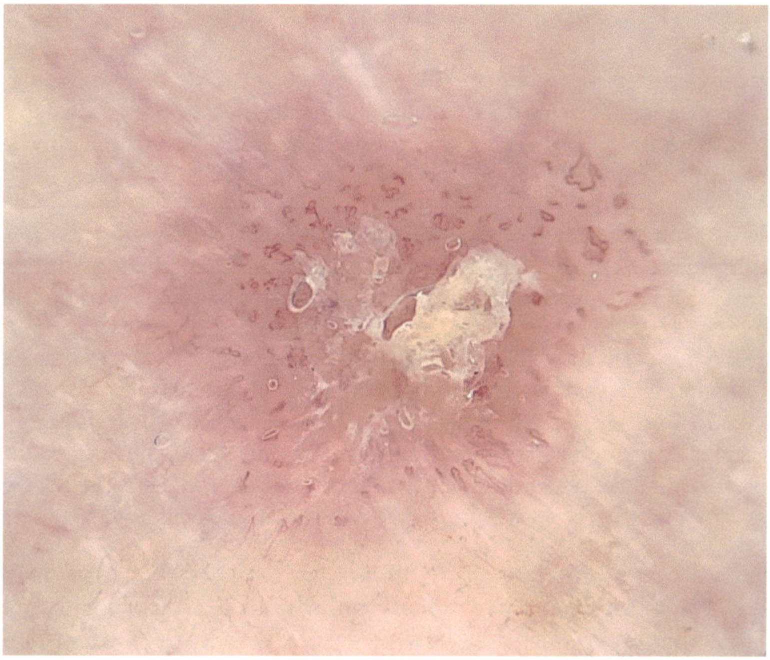

Figure 3.
Dermatoscopic image of bowenoid AK. Dermatoscopically regularly distributed glomerular (upper left) and hairpin (right and lower part) vessels in addition to a central white scale are seen.

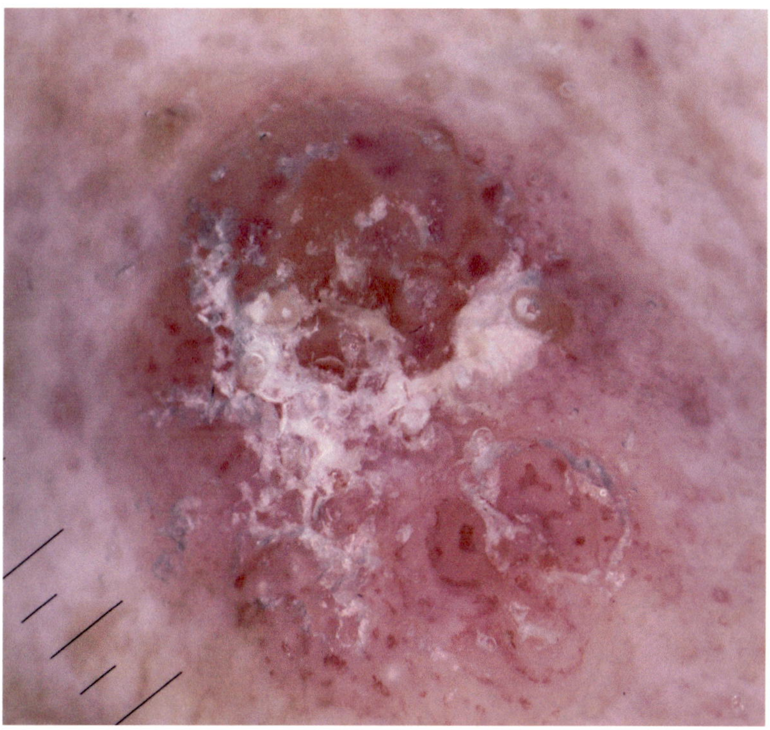

Figure 4.
Dermatoscopic image of bowenoid AK. Dermatoscopically regularly distributed dotted and glomerular vessels, white surface scales, yellow clods corresponding to hyperkeratosis (upper part), and few milia like cysts (lower left fragment) are seen.

3.2.3 Dermatoscopic–histopathologic correlations of AK

Skilled observers can predict the histologic grade of AK with dermatoscopy, although in consensus with clinical features some studies do not find such correlations [37, 38]. The following dermatoscopic–histopathologic correlations have been previously proposed:

- Grade 1 AK on dermatoscopy is typified by a red pseudonetwork and discrete white scales; this pattern correlates with grade I on histopathology where the keratinocytic atypia is mild and limited to the basal and suprabasal layers of the epidermis.
- Grade 2 AK is dermatoscopically characterized by an erythematous background intermingled with white to yellow, keratotic, and enlarged follicular openings. This described pattern in dermatoscopy resembles the surface of a strawberry, therefore was originally termed a strawberry pattern. In grade 2 AK, the histopathological changes are diffuse, with the lower two-thirds of the epidermis involved by atypical keratinocytes with alternating orthokeratosis and parakeratosis on the surface.
- Grade 3 AKs dermatoscopically exhibit either enlarged follicular openings filled with keratotic plugs over a scaly and white-yellow-appearing background or marked hyperkeratosis seen as white-yellow structureless areas. This grade on dermatoscopy corresponds to full-thickness atypia with increased mitotic activity and hyperkeratosis/parakeratosis [39].

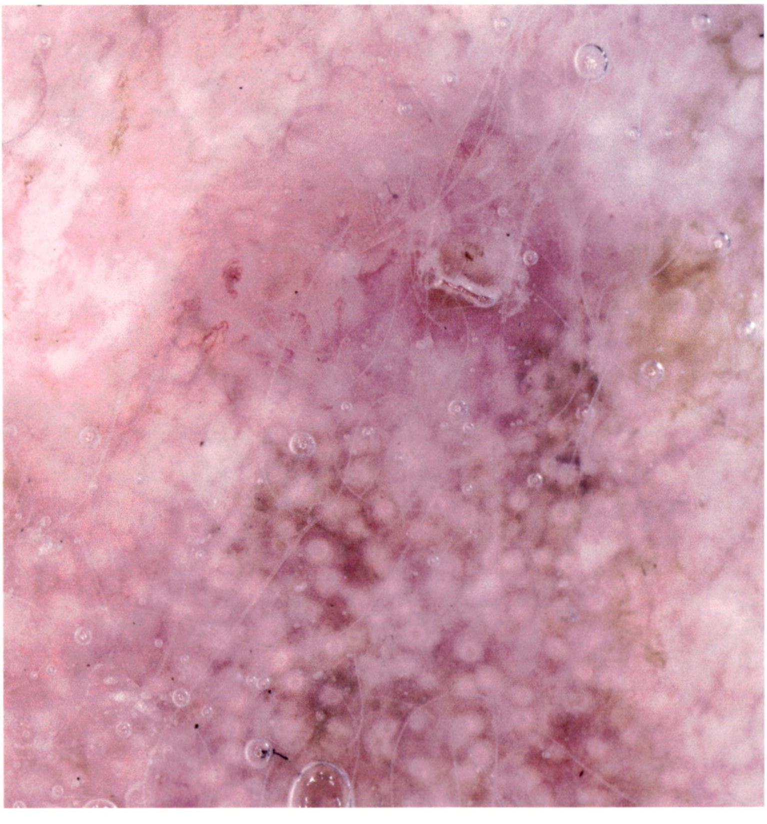

Figure 5.
Histopathologically confirmed basosquamous carcinoma on the border of an AK. Dermatoscopically, two coalescent nodules, both with central ulceration and crust and peripheral dotted and hairpin vessels with white surrounding halo can be seen.

3.3 Dermatoscopic features of AK progressing to SCC

Progression from AK to SCC might follow two pathways. The classical multistep pathway requires proliferation of atypical keratinocytes upwards through the entire epidermis and accumulation of further mutational and cellular events that lead to invasive growth [40]. Nevertheless, the differentiated pathway assumes that invasive SCC may directly arise from a proliferation of atypical basaloid cells of the epidermal basal layer without full-thickness atypia [41].

Dermatoscopic features suggesting progression of AK towards SCC are dotted/glomerular vessels, hairpin vessels, white halos surrounding vessels, ulceration/bleeding, white structureless areas, and white circles surrounding follicles [24]. Appearance of these additional dermatoscopic features is an important clue to perform a diagnostic biopsy even in long-standing AKs, as a great majority of SCCs are associated with preexisting AKs [3] (**Figure 5**).

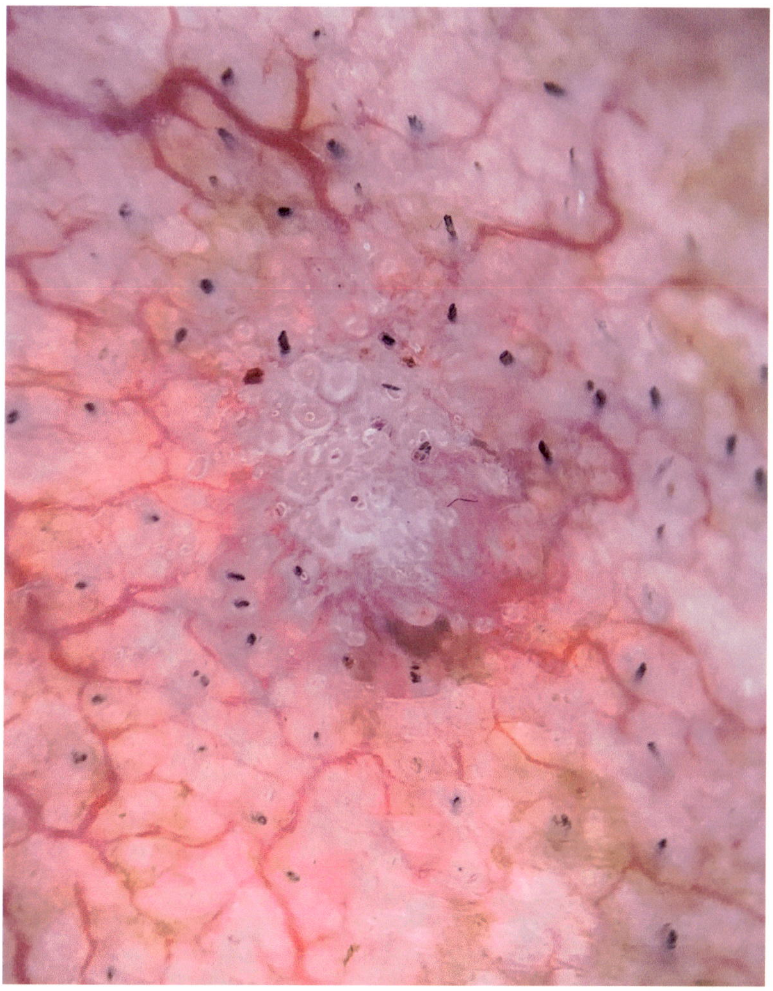

Figure 6.
A lesion on the lower part of the left cheek that clinically presented as an erythematous indurated papule 5 mm in diameter. Dermatoscopically white circles (throughout the lesion), white structureless area (lower part), rosettes (in periphery), and dotted vessels (on the lower part) can be seen. Histopathologically, the basal growth pattern showed filiform papillary elongation protruding into the upper dermal structures in length that exceeds the overlying epidermis.

3.3.1 Characteristics of specific features

3.3.1.1 White circles

On the basis of dermatoscopic–histopathologic correlation, white circles correspond to acanthosis and hypergranulosis of the infundibular epidermis or hyperkeratosis of the infundibular epidermis associated with central keratin plugs [28, 42].

White circles (**Figure 6**) are a specific feature of SCCs and keratoacanthoma-like SCC (KA) and have been shown to be equally common in both and more frequently than in other raised nonpigmented lesions. Moreover, when SCC and KA-like SCC were contrasted with AK and Bowen's disease, the positive predictive value of white circles was 92% in favor of SCC and KA-like SCC [42]. Nevertheless, another study did not find a statistically significant difference between the prevalence of white circles in KA-like SCC and SCC, vs., AK and BD [28]. Other lesions with white circles described are basal cell carcinomas, Bowen's disease, seborrheic keratosis, lichen planus–like keratosis, lichen simplex chronicus, folliculitis, ulcer, chondrodermatitis nodularis helicis, and a dermal nevus [42].

4. Conclusion

Dermatoscopy is a useful tool for the differentiation of AK, IEC, and other non-pigmented facial lesions. The diagnosis is based on the combination of lesion specific factors such as background and follicular structures, vascular patterns, and surface characteristics in addition to information received from the surrounding skin.

Author details

Alise Balcere
Department of Dermatology and Venereology, Riga Stradiņš University, Riga, Latvia

*Address all correspondence to: alise.balcere@gmail.com

References

[1] Zalaudek I, Giacomel J, Schmid K, Bondino S, Rosendahl C, Cavicchini S, et al. Dermatoscopy of facial actinic keratosis, intraepidermal carcinoma, and invasive squamous cell carcinoma: A progression model. J. Am. Acad. Dermatol. 2012;66:589-97. DOI: 10.1016/j.jaad.2011.02.011.

[2] Casari A, Chester J, Pellacani G. Actinic Keratosis and Non-Invasive Diagnostic Techniques: An Update. Biomedicines 2018;6. DOI: 10.3390/biomedicines6010008

[3] Criscione VD, Weinstock MA, Naylor MF, Luque C, Eide MJ, Bingham SF. Actinic keratoses: Natural history and risk of malignant transformation in the veterans affairs topical tretinoin chemoprevention trial. Cancer 2009;115:2523-30. DOI: 10.1002/cncr.24284.

[4] Cassarino DS, DeRienzo DP, Barr RJ. Cutaneous squamous cell carcinoma: A comprehensive clinicopathologic classification - Part two. J. Cutan. Pathol. 2006;33:261-79. DOI: 10.1111/j.0303-6987.2006.00516.x.

[5] Ferrándiz C, Malvehy J, Guillén C, Ferrándiz-Pulido C, Fernández-Figueras M. Precancerous Skin Lesions. Actas Dermosifiliogr. 2017;108:31-41. DOI: 10.1016/j.ad.2016.07.016.

[6] Reinehr CPH, Bakos RM. Actinic keratoses: review of clinical, dermoscopic, and therapeutic aspects. An. Bras. Dermatol. 2019;94(6):637-657. DOI: 10.1016/j.abd.2019.10.0047.

[7] Eisen DB, Asgari MM, Bennett DD, Connolly SM, Dellavalle RP, Freeman EE, et al. Guidelines of care for the management of actinic keratosis. J. Am. Acad. Dermatol. 2021;S0190-9622(21)00502-8. DOI: 10.1016/j.jaad.2021.02.082

[8] Rowert-Huber J, Patel MJ, Forschner T, Ulrich C, Eberle J, Kerl H, et al. Actinic keratosis is an early in situ squamous cell carcinoma: a proposal for reclassification. Br. J. Dermatol. 2007;156:8-12. DOI: 10.1111/j.1365-2133.2007.07860.x.

[9] Inskip M, Cameron A, Akay BN, Gorji M, Clark SP, Rosendahl N, et al. Dermatoscopic features of pigmented intraepidermal carcinoma on the head and neck. JDDG - J. Ger. Soc. Dermatology 2020;18:969-76. DOI: 10.1111/ddg.14220

[10] Conforti C, Dianzani C, Bonin S, Nardon E, Giuffrida R, Di Meo N, et al. Extragenital/extraungueal Bowen disease arising in the absence of field cancerisation is not associated with human papillomavirus infection: Results from a pilot study. Australas. J. Dermatol. 2020;61:e484-6. DOI: 10.1111/ajd.13372

[11] Bhawan J. Squamous cell carcinoma in situ in skin: What does it mean? J. Cutan. Pathol. 2007;34:953-5. DOI: 10.1111/j.1600-0560.2007.00736.x

[12] Murao K, Yoshioka R, Kubo Y. Human papillomavirus infection in Bowen disease: Negative p53 expression, not p16INK4a overexpression, is correlated with human papillomavirus-associated Bowen disease. J. Dermatol. 2014;41:878-84. DOI: 10.1111/1346-8138.12613

[13] Ehrig T, Cockerell C, Piacquadio D, Dromgoole S. Actinic keratoses and the incidence of occult squamous cell carcinoma: A clinical-histopathologic correlation. Dermatologic Surg. 2006;32:1261-5. DOI: 10.1111/j.1524-4725.2006.32287.x

[14] Buinauskaite E, Makstiene J, Buinauskiene J, Valiukeviciene S. Reliability of solar keratosis clinical

diagnosis: A prospective study. Australas. J. Dermatol. 2015;56:e49–e52. DOI: 10.1111/ajd.12095

[15] Valdés-Morales KL, Peralta-Pedrero ML, Jurado-Santa Cruz F, Morales-Sanchez MA. Diagnostic Accuracy of Dermoscopy of Actinic Keratosis: A Systematic Review. Dermatol. Pract. Concept. 2020;10:e20200121. DOI: 10.5826/dpc.1004a121

[16] Huerta-Brogeras M, Olmos O, Borbujo J, Hernández-Núñez A, Castaño E, Romero-Maté A, et al. Validation of dermoscopy as a real-time noninvasive diagnostic imaging technique for actinic keratosis. Arch. Dermatol. 2012;148:1159-64. DOI: 10.1001/archdermatol.2012.1060

[17] Warszawik-Hendzel O, Olszewska M, Maj M, Rakowska A, Czuwara J, Rudnicka L. Non-invasive diagnostic techniques in the diagnosis of squamous cell carcinoma. J. Dermatol. Case Rep. 2015;9:89-97. DOI: 10.3315/jdcr.2015.1221

[18] Pyne JH, Myint E, Clark SP, Clifopoulos C, Fishburn P, Gorji M, et al. Squamous cell carcinoma: pain as a clue to increased tumour diameter, increased invasion depth, the grade of differentiation, acantholysis and perineural invasion. Clin. Exp. Dermatol. 2020;45:180-6. DOI: 10.1111/ced.14066

[19] Olsen EA, Lisa Abernethy M, Kulp-Shorten C, Callen JP, Glazer SD, Huntley A, et al. A double-blind, vehicle-controlled study evaluating masoprocol cream in the treatment of actinic keratoses on the head and neck. J. Am. Acad. Dermatol. 1991;24 (5 Pt 1):738-743. DOI: 10.1016/0190-9622(91)70113-g

[20] Schmitz L, Kahl P, Majores M, Bierhoff E, Stockfleth E, Dirschka T. Actinic keratosis: correlation between clinical and histological classification systems. J. Eur. Acad. Dermatology Venereol. 2016;30:1303-7. DOI: 10.1111/jdv.13626

[21] Yélamos O, Braun RP, Liopyris K, Wolner ZJ, Kerl K, Gerami P, et al. Dermoscopy and dermatopathology correlates of cutaneous neoplasms. J. Am. Acad. Dermatol. 2019;80:341-63. DOI: 10.1016/j.jaad.2018.07.073

[22] Kittler H, Marghoob AA, Argenziano G, Carrera C, Curiel-Lewandrowski C, Hofmann-Wellenhof R, et al. Standardization of terminology in dermoscopy/dermatoscopy: Results of the third consensus conference of the International Society of Dermoscopy. J. Am. Acad. Dermatol. 2016;74(6):1093-1106. DOI: 10.1016/j.jaad.2015.12.038

[23] Zalaudek I, Giacomel J, Argenziano G, Hofmann-Wellenhof R, Micantonio T, Di Stefani A, et al. Dermoscopy of facial nonpigmented actinic keratosis. Br. J. Dermatol. 2006;155:951-6. DOI: 10.1111/j.1365-2133.2006.07426.x

[24] Papageorgiou C, Lallas A, Manoli SM, Longo C, Lai M, Liopyris K, et al. Evaluation of dermatoscopic criteria for early detection of squamous cell carcinoma arising on an actinic keratosis. J. Am. Acad. Dermatol. 2021;S0190-9622(21)00760-X. DOI: 10.1016/j.jaad.2021.03.111

[25] Balagula Y, Braun RP, Rabinovitz HS, Dusza SW, Scope A, Liebman TN, et al. The significance of crystalline/chrysalis structures in the diagnosis of melanocytic and nonmelanocytic lesions. J. Am. Acad. Dermatol. 2012;67:194.e1-194.e8. DOI: 10.1016/j.jaad.2011.04.039

[26] Tschandl P, Rinner C, Apalla Z, Argenziano G, Codella N, Halpern A, et al. Human–computer collaboration for skin cancer recognition. Nat Med.

2020;26(8):1229-1234. DOI: 10.1038/s41591-020-0942-0

[27] Mir-Bonafé JF, Rozas-Muñoz E, Dalmau J, Mir-Bonafé M, Iznardo H, García-Melendo C, et al. Iceberg sign as a dermoscopic clue of actinic keratosis neglecta. J. Eur. Acad. Dermatology Venereol. 2019;33:e254-6. DOI: 10.1111/jdv.15484

[28] Ertop Doğan P, Akay BN, Okçu Heper A, Rosendahl C, Erdem C. Dermatoscopic findings and dermatopathological correlates in clinical variants of actinic keratosis, Bowen's disease, keratoacanthoma, and squamous cell carcinoma. Dermatol. Ther. 2021;1-9. DOI: 10.1111/dth.14877

[29] Haspeslagh M, Noë M, De Wispelaere I, Degryse N, Vossaert K, Lanssens S, et al. Rosettes and other white shiny structures in polarized dermoscopy: Histological correlate and optical explanation. J. Eur. Acad. Dermatology Venereol. 2016;30(2):311-313. DOI: 10.1111/jdv.13080

[30] Balcere A, Ozola E, Karls R, Čēma I, Rone Kupfere M, Krūmiņa A. Dermoscopic monitoring of shiny white streaks during topical treatment of actinic keratosis. In: Proceedings of the 62nd International Scientific Conference of Daugavpils University. 2020. page 139-43.

[31] Pizzichetta MA, Canzonieri V, Soyer PH, Rubegni P, Talamini R, Massone C. Negative Pigment Network and Shiny White Streaks. Am. J. Dermatopathol. 2014;36(5):433-438. DOI: 10.1097/DAD.0000000000000019

[32] Conforti C, Giuffrida R, Pizzichetta MA, Di Meo N, Magaton-Rizzi G, Zalaudek I. Integrating the concept of field cancerization in the classification and risk assessment of cutaneous squamous cell carcinoma: proposal for a new classification and terminology of keratinocyte skin cancer. J. Eur. Acad. Dermatology Venereol. 2019;33:e327-30. DOI: 10.1111/jdv.15624

[33] Martín JM, Bella-Navarro R, Jordá E. Vascular patterns in dermoscopy. Actas Dermosifiliogr. 2012;103:357-75. DOI: 10.1016/j.ad.2011.11.005

[34] Yang Y, Lin J, Fang S, Han S, Song Z. What's new in dermoscopy of Bowen's disease: two new dermoscopic signs and its differential diagnosis. Int. J. Dermatol. 2017;56:1022-5. DOI: 10.1111/ijd.13734

[35] Pan Y, Chamberlain AJ, Bailey M, Chong AH, Haskett M, Kelly JW. Dermatoscopy aids in the diagnosis of the solitary red scaly patch or plaque-features distinguishing superficial basal cell carcinoma, intraepidermal carcinoma, and psoriasis. J. Am. Acad. Dermatol. 2008;59:268-74. DOI: 10.1016/j.jaad.2008.05.013

[36] Karaali MG, Polat AK, Sarı Y, Aksu AEK, Leblebici C, Gurel MS. Proliferative actinic keratosis: An invasive squamous cell carcinoma or not? Acta Dermatovenerologica Croat. 2019;27:75-80.

[37] Lee DW, Kim DY, Hong JH, Seo SH, Kye YC, Ahn HH. Correlations between histopathologic and dermoscopic findings in Korean actinic keratosis. Microsc. Res. Tech. 2019;82(1):12-17. DOI: 10.1002/jemt.23043

[38] Longo M, Arias-Santiago S, de las Heras E, Fernandez-Guarino M, Lopez-Estebaranz JL, Toll A, et al. Clinical and dermatoscopic evaluation and degree of dysplasia of actinic keratoses: Differences among skin cancer experts. J. Am. Acad. Dermatol. 2015;72:AB182. DOI: 10.1016/j.jaad.2015.02.742

[39] Zalaudek I, Piana S, Moscarella E, Longo C, Zendri E, Castagnetti F, et al. Morphologic grading and treatment of

facial actinic keratosis. Clin. Dermatol. 2014;32:80-7. DOI: 10.1016/j.clindermatol.2013.05.028.

[40] Stratigos A, Garbe C, Lebbe C, Malvehy J, Del Marmol V, Pehamberger H, et al. Diagnosis and treatment of invasive squamous cell carcinoma of the skin: European consensus-based interdisciplinary guideline. Eur. J. Cancer 2015;51:1989-2007. DOI: 10.1016/j.ejca.2015.06.110

[41] Fernández-Figueras MT, Carrato C, Sáenz X, Puig L, Musulen E, Ferrándiz C, et al. Actinic keratosis with atypical basal cells (AK I) is the most common lesion associated with invasive squamous cell carcinoma of the skin. J. Eur. Acad. Dermatology Venereol. 2015;29:991-7. DOI: 10.1111/jdv.12848

[42] Rosendahl C, Cameron A, Argenziano G, Zalaudek I, Tschandl P, Kittler H. Dermoscopy of squamous cell carcinoma and keratoacanthoma. Arch. Dermatol. 2012;148(12):1386-1392. DOI: 10.1001/archdermatol.2012.2974

Section 3

Melanocytic Lesions

Chapter 4

Combined Nevi

Jelena Stojkovic-Filipovic and Miljan Vlahovic

Abstract

Combined nevi (CN) are clinically defined as melanocytic lesions comprising two or more distinct melanocytic nevus components, and from the cytological point of view, CN are determined by the presence of two or more different nevus cell types in one biopsy specimen. They are very uncommon and represent less than 1% of all biopsied melanocytic nevi. CN comprise any melanocytic nevi, but the most prevalent combination is CN that consist of blue nevus associated with common melanocytic nevus. CN owe their diversity to combination of different nevi, that are variously combined. Consequently, they can have variable clinical aspects and dermatoscopic features. Because of the presence of at least two distinct subtypes of nevomelanocytes, dermatoscopically CN can show multicomponent, unspecific, and peculiar patterns. Therefore, CN can mimic melanomas, their most important differential clinical, dermatoscopical and histopathological diagnosis.

Keywords: combined nevi, combined blue nevi, melanoma, dermatoscopy, dermoscopy

1. Introduction

Combined nevi (CN) are specific, uncommon type of melanocytic nevi, and they represent less than 1% of all biopsied melanocytic nevi [1, 2]. Clinically, they are defined as melanocytic lesions comprising two or more distinct melanocytic nevus components [3]. From a histopathologic point of view, combined nevi are determined by the presence of two or more different nevus cell types in one biopsy specimen [4]. Based on their clinical and histopathological features, CN represent a subcategory of so-called collision or compound tumors, which are defined by the occurrence of two distinctive neoplastic skin lesions, that collide concurrently within the same specimen [5].

Combined nevi can be comprised by any melanocytic nevi. Although any collision is possible, it is most likely that CN present a combined variant of blue nevus, acquired nevus (Clark nevus), superficial congenital nevus, Spitz nevus or deep penetrating nevus [1]. The most frequent combination that is seen in practice is that of blue nevus associated with common melanocytic nevus and Spitz nevus [4].

2. Clinical features

Combined nevi are mainly congenital, although they are not always visible at birth, but later in life [6]. Although CN could be seen in childhood, as well as at an old age, they are most frequent in young adults (median age reported from 29 to 47) [1, 4, 7, 8]. In early studies of CN, a slight predominance in females was reported

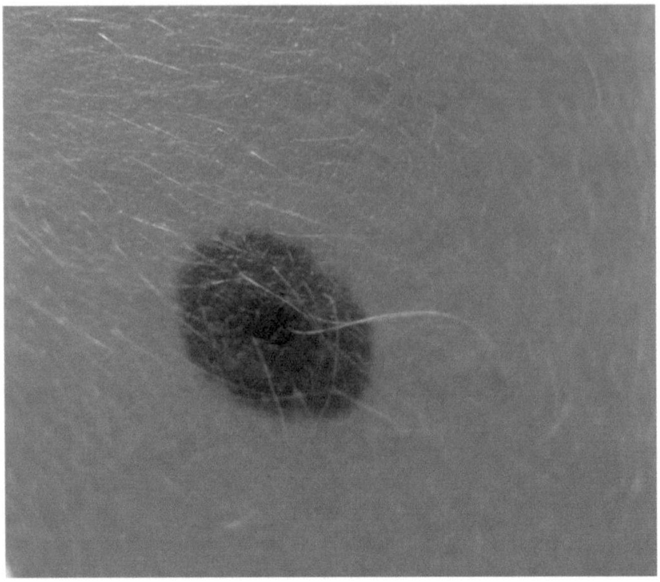

Figure 1.
Combined nevus clinical presentation: Slightly raised, round lesion; small black spot in the center, surrounded by brown area (Targetoid combined blue nevus type).

[1, 4, 8], with the female: male ratio 1.1:1 [1]. Newer study with larger number of observed CN, has shifted that ratio towards male predominance 0.6:1 [7].

In the view of distribution, the predilection site has not been officially established, but literature data show that this nevus type does most frequently appear on the trunk [1, 4, 7–9] and head and neck region [7], and it is less common on the extremities [7].

Since CN are composed of distinct nevi, their clinical appearance could be very diverse. In practice, CN are usually small, flat, or minimally raised lesions [1, 7], often characterized by a small blue or black spot (corresponding to the blue nevus component) in the context of a larger area of brown color (corresponding to the common nevus) surrounding the blue nevus part [10] (**Figure 1**). The latter is known as the targetoid combined blue nevus type [11].

3. Dermatoscopic features

Since CN are composed of at least two different nevus types in various combinations, their dermatoscopic features are characterized by mostly multicomponent, unspecific, and random patterns. Typically, multicomponent structure of CN exhibit reasonably symmetrical appearance [3, 7] (**Figure 2**), which is consistent with already established findings that benign nevi tend to exhibit symmetry [12]. This is one of the most distinguishing features when differentiating CN from melanomas, as chaos (asymmetry of structure or colors) is principally imperative of a malignant neoplasm [6, 13].

Looking at the color, simultaneous occurrence of different colors (primarily brown and blue, rarely black, and white) is common appearance in CN, where the pigmentation originates from both junctional and dermal portion of the skin [6]. Since blue nevus is the most common component of CN, structureless blue part of the lesion is frequently presented [7], usually covering about 30% of the lesion (**Figure 2A** and **B**). Being such a regular finding, structureless blue area is an important element in the dermatoscopic analysis of this nevus type [7], even

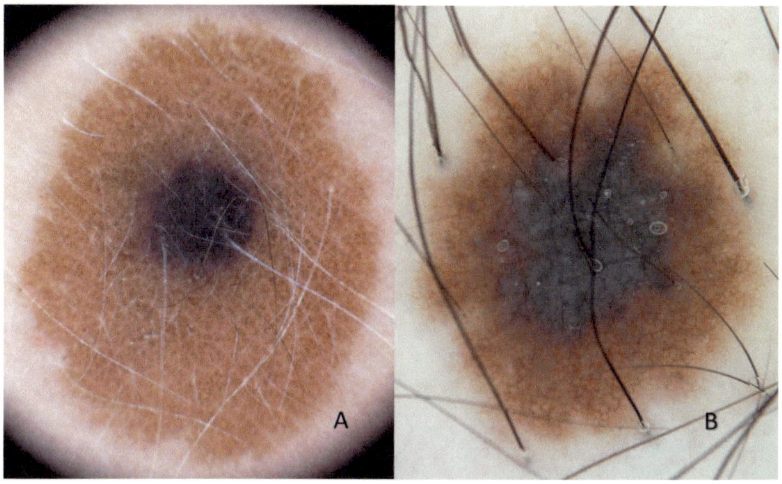

Figure 2.
Combined nevus dermatoscopy: A. well defined structureless blue area in the center of the lesion, pigmented globules at the periphery; B. ill-defined structureless blue area in the center of the lesion, brown reticular lines at the periphery.

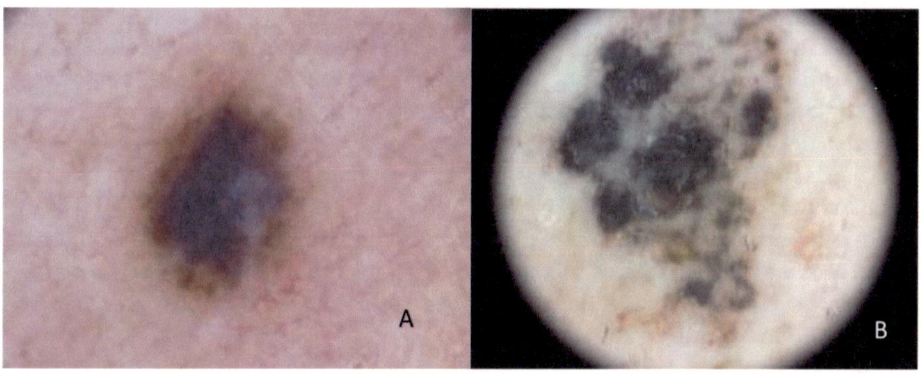

Figure 3.
Combined nevus dermatoscopy: A. diffuse distribution of structureless blue area, structureless brown at the periphery; B. patchy distribution of structureless blue area.

reported as a hallmark of CN [14]. Both well and ill-defined structureless blue areas (**Figure 2A** and **B**) are presented in CN. It is important to remember that the presence of ill-defined structureless blue area in any lesion must always raise suspicion, since it may resemble the "blue veil", common characteristic of melanomas with the blue part [7].

Regarding the position of the structureless blue areas and their proximity to the edge of the lesion, in the majority of observed cases, these areas do not touch the edge of the lesions (**Figure 2A** and **B**) [7]. Diffuse and patchy type of structureless blue areas distribution appears in only less then 10% CN and cannot be considered as a specific feature for this nevus type (**Figure 3A** and **B**). Structureless blue area could be presented either eccentrically (**Figure 4**) or in the central part of CN, whereas central distribution is more common (**Figure 2A** and **B**) [7, 9], distinctive for benign lesions and reflects benign nature of these nevi. If located centrally, blue structureless area is surrounded by another pattern, mostly brown clods (**Figure 2A**), or reticular pattern (**Figure 2B**), which was previously stated as the stereotypical appearance of CN [15]. Within and around the structureless blue area of CN brown

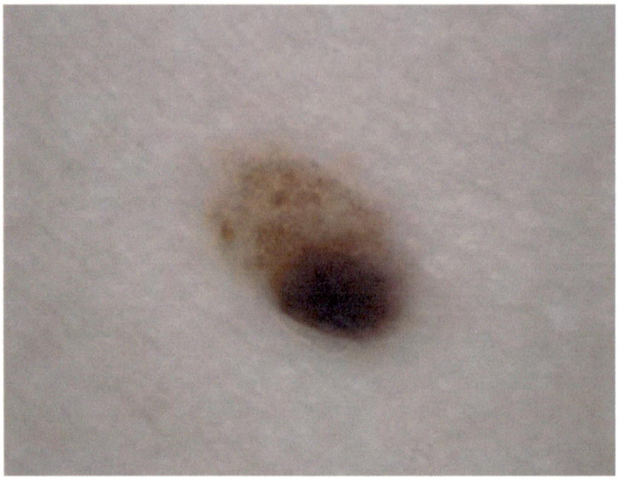

Figure 4.
Combined nevus dermatoscopy: Eccentric structureless blue area, at the edge of the lesion.

dots may be present [14, 16]. Yet, this cannot be considered as a dermatoscopic clue specific for CN, since it could be found in melanomas as well.

Curved lines at the periphery of the lesion can be contemplated as additional specific dermatoscopic features of CN [9, 14]. The other dermatoscopic features like radial circumferential or segmental lines, branched lines, as well as blue and gray clods and dots are not specific for CN [7, 17]. In some cases, when blue nevus is associated with a dermal nevus, gray-blue pigmentation could be distributed irregularly [9].

In cases where CN exhibit chaotic appearance, featuring eccentric structureless, particularly blue area (**Figure 4**), CN lack clues such as white lines, gray structures, pseudopods/radial lines, thick reticular lines, ulcerations, and polygons which are typical for melanomas [7]. Lesions with multicomponent pattern and eccentric, particularly structureless blue area, lacking specific dermatoscopic features of melanoma do not require excision.

4. Differential diagnosis

Due to their variable nature and different nevus types combined in variety of patterns, clinical and dermoscopic determination of CN could be challenging. For that reason, differential diagnoses may include several benign or malignant neoplasms. Combined nevus may resemble blue nevus, common nevus, Spitz nevus (pigmented type), pigmented spindle cell nevus, plexiform spindle cell nevus, benign vascular tumors, hemosiderotic variant of dermatofibroma, pigmented basal cell carcinoma, cutaneous metastases [6, 9, 18, 19]. Despite this broad similarity to the various skin lesions, CN usually simulate melanoma, which is the most common differential diagnosis. Due to their inconsistent, atypical and irregular clinical and dermatoscopic appearance, CN are frequently misdiagnosed as melanomas [1] and careful histologic examination to exclude melanoma is occasionally required.

5. Histopathology

The term "combined" can be both used in cytological and dermatoscopic context. Histopathological features of CN depend on nevi that are combined within the lesion, and vary depending on the nevi types present.

Histopathologically, there are several types of CN, characterized by the combination of any morphological expression of congenital and/or acquired nevi. Superficial congenital nevus combined with blue nevus, either common or cellular type are most common combination seen in practice. Less frequent are Spitz nevus combined with Clark nevus ("SPARK"), superficial congenital nevi combined with deep penetrating nevus, and blue nevus combined with Spitz nevus ("BLITZ") [7].

The most common histopathological finding in diagnosis of CN is a compound or dermal nevus with a dermal population of enlarged nevus cells (**Figure 5A**), either admixed with or overlie pigmented epithelioid and/or spindled melanocytes component in association with melanophages [19] (**Figure 5B** and **C**).

In the case of blue nevus, dendritic, cellular blue or deep penetrating nevus are present, with melanin in the deeper dermal portions [1]. Common blue nevus is characterized by elongated, often slightly wavy melanocytes with long, branching dendrites, either grouped together or in bundles in the upper and mid dermis, parallel to the epidermis, with variable numbers of macrophages and increase amount of collagen [1]. Melanocytes could extend into the subcutaneous tissue or approach the epidermis, but they never alter the epidermis structure [1, 19]. In case of cellular

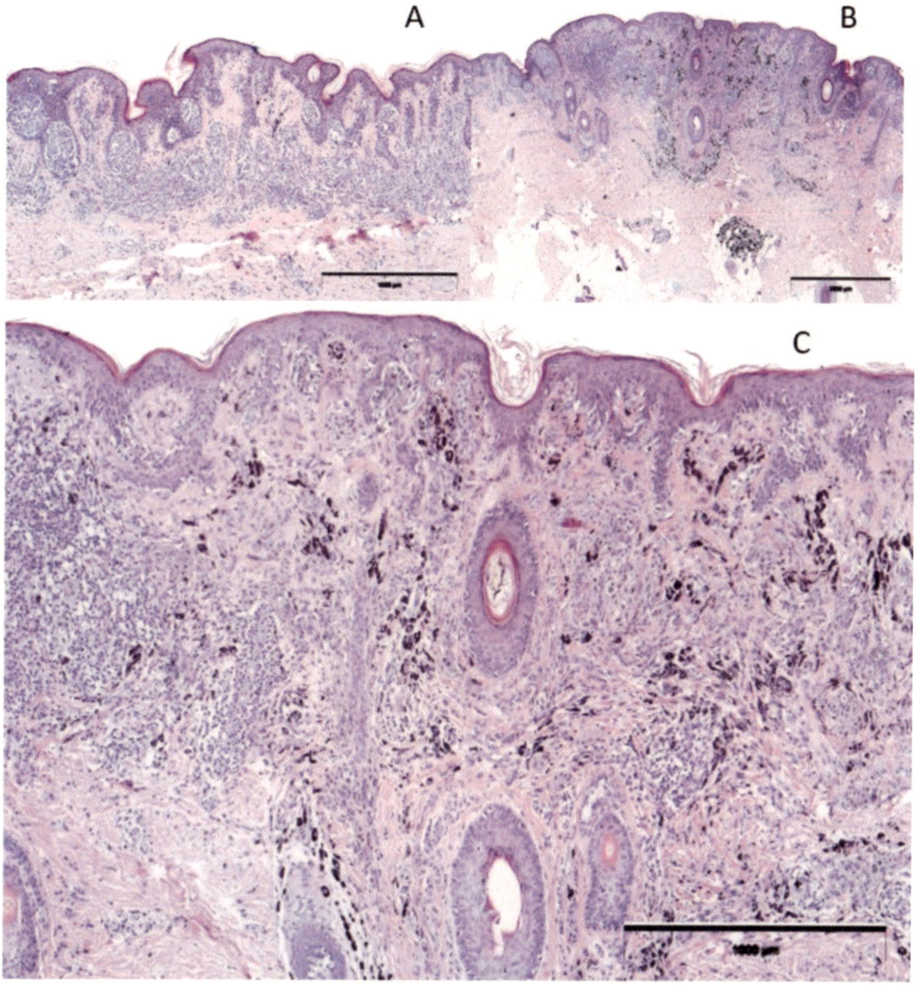

Figure 5.
Combined nevus histopathological findings: A. epidermal and dermal nests of common melanocytic nevus, no signs of atypia or mitotic activity: B, C. slender spindle cells and melanophages in the center of the lesion.

blue nevus, deeply pigmented dendritic melanocytes are visible in addition to nests and fascicles of spindle-shaped cells with abundant pale cytoplasm containing little or no melanin. These melanocytes also frequently penetrate the subcutaneous tissue. Some of the cells may appear atypical, with nuclear pleomorphism accompanied by multinucleated giant cells, rare mitoses, and inflammatory infiltrates. In addition to this, overlapping features of common and cellular blue nevi could be seen in some lesions [19].

If Spitz nevus is present, nests of large epithelioid cells, spindle cells or both can be seen, usually extending from the epidermis into the reticular dermis, within hyperplastic epidermis and mononuclear and multinucleate giant epithelioid cells infiltrating dermal collagen. In some observed cases, necrotic cells, mitotic figures and intraepidermal eosinophilic globules were found [19].

6. Management

Better and more uniformed description of clinical and dermatoscopic features of CN, together with improvement in routine differentiation between CN and melanomas can significantly reduce the number of excisions and biopsies performed. Biopsy should still be considered for any suspicious lesion. If distinction from melanoma cannot be clearly made, complete surgical excision is recommended.

Author details

Jelena Stojkovic-Filipovic[1,2*] and Miljan Vlahovic[3,4]

1 Clinic of Dermatovnereology, University Clinical Center of Serbia, Belgrade, Serbia

2 Faculty of Medicine, University of Belgrade, Belgrade, Serbia

3 Department of Health NSW, Sydney, NSW, Australia

4 Monash University, Melbourne, VIC, Australia

*Address all correspondence to: sf.jelena@gmail.com

References

[1] Scolyer RA, Zhuang L, Palmer AA, Thompson JF, McCarthy SW. Combined naevus: a benign lesion frequently misdiagnosed both clinically and pathologically as melanoma. Pathology. 2004;36(5):419-27

[2] Strungs I. Common and uncommon variants of melanocytic naevi. Pathology. 2004;36(5):396-403

[3] Barnhill RL. Combined naevus. In: LeBoitPE, Burg G, Weedon D, Sarasin A, eds. World Health Organization Classification of Tumours Pathology & Genetics Skin Tumours. Lyon: IARC Press, 2006; 100-102

[4] Baran JL, Duncan LM. Combined melanocytic nevi: histologic variants and melanoma mimics. Am J Surg Pathol. 2011;35:1540-8.

[5] Cosme Alvarez Cuesta C, Vazquez Lopez F, Perez Oliva N. Dermatoscopy in the diagnosis of cutaneous collision. Clin Exp Dermatol 2004;29:199-200.

[6] Kittler H, editor. Dermatoscopy. Pattern analysis of pigmented and non-pigmented lesions. Vienna: Facultas Universitatsverlag, 2nd edition. 2016.

[7] J. Stojkovic-Filipovic, D. Tiodorovic, A. Lallas, et al. Dermatoscopy of combined blue nevi: a multicentre study of the International Dermoscopy Society. JEADV 2020;....: 900-905

[8] Schweizer A, Fink C, Bertlich I et al. Differentiation of combined nevi and melanomas: Case-control study with comparative analysis of dermoscopic features. J Dtsch Dermatol Ges. 2020;18:111-118.).

[9] de Giorgi V, Massi D, Salvini C et al. Dermoscopic features of combined melanocytic nevi. J Cutan Pathol. 2004;31:600-4.

[10] Dermoscopy of melanocytic neoplasms: combined blue nevi. Arch Dermatol. 2004;140:902.

[11] Argenziano G. Dermoscopy of melanocytic neoplasms: Targetoid combined blue nevi. Arch Dermatol. 2004;140:1576.

[12] Kim JK, Nelson KC. Dermoscopic features of common nevi: a review. G Ital Dermatol Venereol. 2012;147(2):141-8.

[13] Rosendahl C, Cameron A, McColl I, Wilkinson D. Dermatoscopy in routine practice – 'chaos and clues'. Aust Fam Physician. 2012;41:482-7.

[14] Ferrari A, Lozzi GP, Fargnoli MC, Peris K. Dermoscopic evolution of a congenital combined nevus in childhood. Dermatol Surg. 2005;31 (11 Pt 1):1448-50.

[15] Zalaudek I, Manzo M, Savarese I et al. The morphologic universe of melanocytic nevi. Semin Cutan Med Surg. 2009;28:149-56.

[16] Piccolo D, Altamura D, Lozzi GP, Peris K. Blue-whitish veil-like structure as the primary dermoscopic feature of combined nevus. Dermatol Surg. 2006;321176-8.

[17] Yaginuma A, Nobeyama Y, Miyake-Nakano S et al. Case of combined nevus showing a speckled distribution pattern. J Dermatol. 2018;45:e232-e233

[18] Cabo H. Combined nevi. In H. P. Soyer, G. Argenziano, R. Hofmann-Wellenhof, R. H. Johr (Eds.). Color Atlas of Melanocytic Lesions of the Skin. Springer. 2007; 97-101.

[19] Bolognia J, Scaffer JV, Cerroni L. Dermatology. St Louis: Mosby Elsevier; 2018.

Section 4

Special Sites

Chapter 5

Pigmented Lesions of the Eyelid Margin

Wojciech Adamski and Kinga Adamska

Abstract

The eyelid area poses a diagnostic and therapeutic challenge due to its specific anatomy. The eyelid is composed of skin, orbicularis muscle, tarsus, and the eyelid margin is continuous with palpebral conjunctiva. Among pigmented tumors, benign lesions such as epidermal or intradermal nevi, freckles, lentigo, or seborrheic keratosis are the most common. Melanoma is relatively rare in this location. A suspicious lesion may be biopsied or excised. Surgery in the eyelid area requires special considerations to maintain a safe surgical margin, vital function of the eyelid, and acceptable cosmetic effect due to the exposure of the eyelid region of the face.

Keywords: eyelid, margin, nevus, melanoma, seborrheic keratosis

1. Introduction

The main functions of the eyelid are to provide protection for the moist surface of the eye. Due to its function and exposition to outside factors such as sunlight, it has distinctive anatomy and requires a unique approach. Because of its location

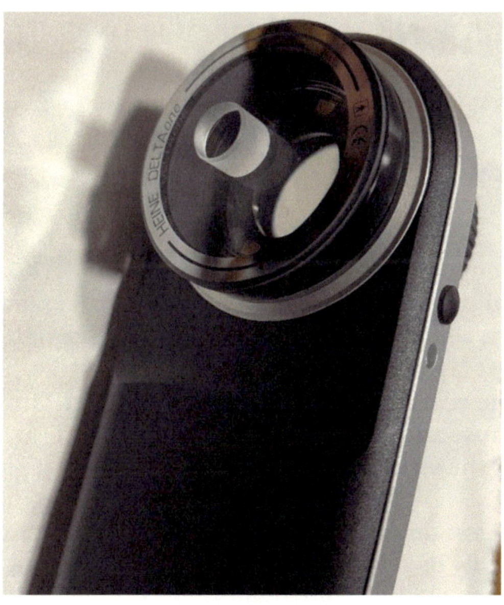

Figure 1.
A hand dermatoscope with a contact plate designed for difficult anatomical locations.

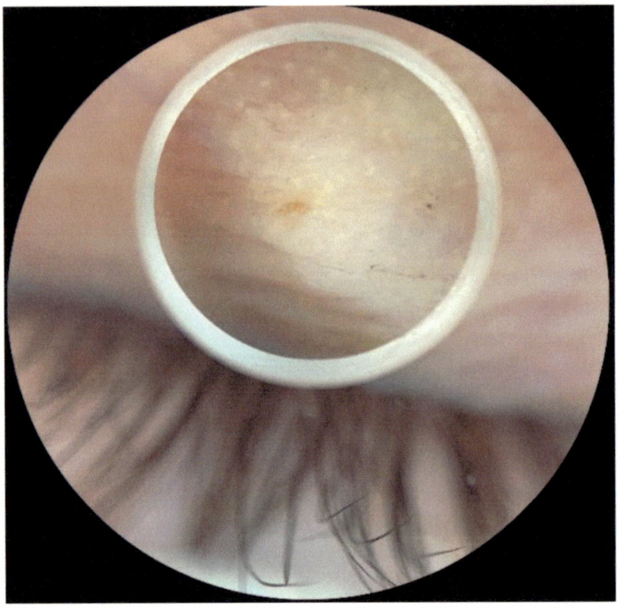

Figure 2.
A small junctional nevus visualized with a contact plate designed for difficult locations.

and morphology, it often poses a challenge for contact dermatoscopy in diagnosis and requires distinct surgical methods when such an approach is necessary. Lesions located in the eyelid area may be visualized using a non-contact dermatoscope. More accessible areas of this region may be visualized with contact dermatoscopy using a non-alcoholic medium and a special contact plate designed to be used in difficult anatomical locations (**Figures 1** and **2**). Due to a close relation with sensitive conjunctiva, the examination may be preceded by applying local anesthetic drop (e.g. Proxymetacainum) into the conjunctival sack in order to prevent pain reflex and eyelid closure. To reduce the risk of irritation, an ophthalmic gel may be used instead of the immersion fluid. Another less recommended approach may involve a dry dermatoscopy, without a contact plate or with a contact plate, but without immersion fluid.

2. Relevant anatomy

The eyelid can be divided into four layers. Eyelid skin is continuous with the skin of the face, although it is substantially thinner. Underneath the skin lies the striated muscle called the orbicularis muscle, which is responsible for eye closure. Deeper lies the tarsus, a strong plate of dense connective tissue with meibomian glands. The innermost layer of the eyelid is the conjunctiva. The eyelids contain various glands like the eccrine sweat glands of the eyelid skin and the accessory lacrimal gland of Krause and Wolfring in the conjunctiva, the gland of Moll (an apocrine gland), and the sebaceous glands–the Meibomian glands and the glands of Zeiss.

Benign and malignant tumors may originate in all of the mentioned layers, although they are usually of skin origin, mostly epidermal [1].

Although the most numerous epithelial tumors of the eyelid margin like basal cell carcinoma except for its pigmented variant, epithelial cysts, or actinic keratosis will mainly not be discussed in this chapter.

3. Benign melanocytic eyelid tumors

3.1 Freckles

Freckles are small (1–5 mm in diameter), flat brown skin spots located in skin exposed to sunlight. They are usually multiple lesions in one site. Histologically, there is hyperpigmentation of the basal cell layer but no elongation of the rete ridges. They tend to darken after exposition to sunlight and lighten when devoid of it. With time they may clinically disappear. Dermoscopic features include evenly distributed pigmentation and a moth-eaten border [2, 3].

3.2 Simple lentigo

Simple lentigo (lentigo simplex) is a skin lesion with well-demarcated borders, light to dark brown. Arise due to melanocyte proliferation in the basal layer of the epidermis. They do not darken when exposed to sunlight which differentiates them from freckles. Multiple appearances of lentigo simplex lesions are called lentiginosis [4]. Dermatoscopic features include structureless homogenous pigmentation. These lesions may be congenital and may be associated with genetic syndromes like Peutz-Jeghers Syndrome, Carney Complex, or LEOPARD Syndrome [5]. Dermatoscopic features include a uniform thin brown, black or blue network (**Figures 3** and **4**).

3.3 Nevi

Nevus is commonly found in the area of the eyelids. It is a heterogeneous group of lesions with a wide array of clinical and histological presentation.

3.4 Congenital nevus

A congenital nevus is found in the skin of the eyelids in about 1% of newborns. It may vary in size, from small to large. Large lesions have a higher rate of malignant transformation. Histologically a congenital nevus is similar to an acquired nevus.

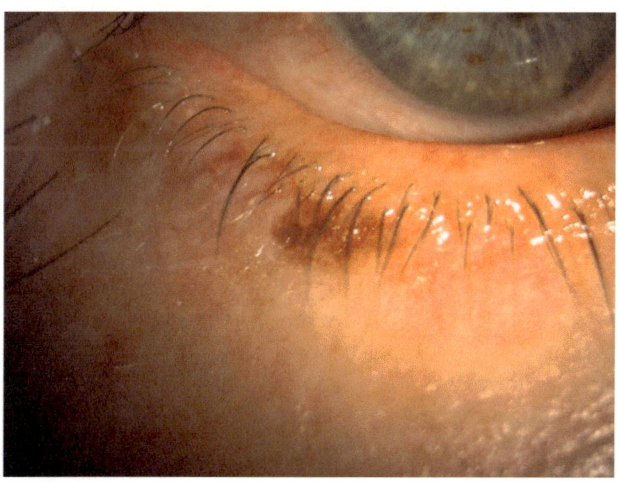

Figure 3.
Lentigo simplex of the lower eyelid.

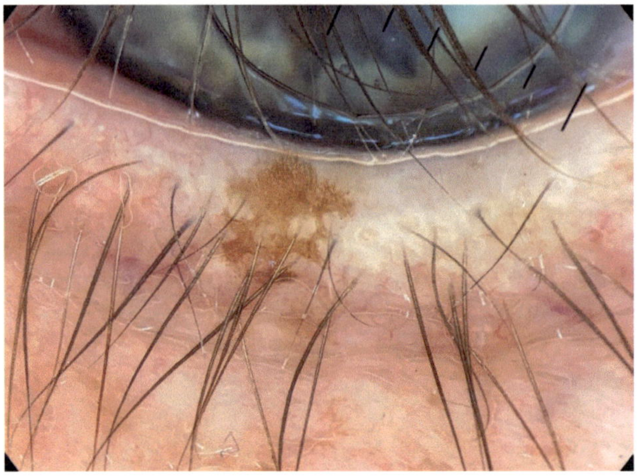

Figure 4.
Lentigo.

3.5 Kissing nevus

A kissing or split nevus is a rare subtype of a congenital nevus that appear on both the upper and lower eyelid. Its unique morphology indicates that it developed early in utero, before the 20th week of gestation, when the eyelids are divided [6, 7]. Due to its difficult location involving both eyelids and usually a large diameter as well as typically benign nature, those type of nevi are not usually surgically treated [7].

3.6 Nevus of Ota

Nevus of Ota (oculodermal melanocytosis) is a benign melanocytic lesion involving the face and eyelid region, specifically the area supported by the ophthalmic and maxillary branches of the trigeminal nerve. It is usually congenital but may appear in puberty. It appears due to the entrapment of melanocytes in the upper third of the dermis. The deeper location of melanocytes gives this lesion a blue/gray appearance. The cause of the failure of migration of the melanocytes to their typical location in the basal layer of the epidermis remains unknown. In addition to covering the eyelids nevus of Ota may also involve the conjunctiva as well as the sclera, increasing the risk of developing glaucoma. It also affects the uveal tract of the eye, increasing the risk of uveal melanoma. Histologically distinct dendritic melanocytes can be found in the affected areas [8]. It is usually unilateral. Some authors use the term "nevus of Hori" for a bilateral involvement [9].

3.7 Acquired nevus

Acquired nevus appears commonly in the eyelid area. The lesions usually appear in childhood and may increase in size during patient growth.

Histologically there are three main types of acquired nevus, according to the location of melanocyte proliferation: the junctional nevus, located in the dermo-epidermal junction, the intradermal nevus, located only in the dermis, and the compound nevus, which involves both of these locations. Junctional appears mainly among younger patients and presents as a flat, evenly colored spot. Dermatoscopic features include reticular or globular patterns, interrupted by the presence of follicular openings, the intradermal nevus is located deeper in the dermis and may be elevated or papillomatous in shape. It might be slightly pigmented or have no pigmentation (achromic) at all. Dermatoscopic features may include comma vessels, globular pattern, centered coma, and occasionally arborizing vessels in case of repetitive trauma. A compound nevus combines the characteristics of the previous lesions.

A distinct subtype of intradermal nevus appearing in the face and neck region is called the Miescher's nevus. Its dermatoscopic features may include a homogeneous globular pattern with the focal and symmetric arrangement of globules arranged in a cobblestone pattern.

Some achromic intradermal nevus located on the eyelid margin may be misdiagnosed as basal cell carcinoma, which is typically found in the lower eyelid. Madarosis is often associated as a sign of malignancy, brown structureless

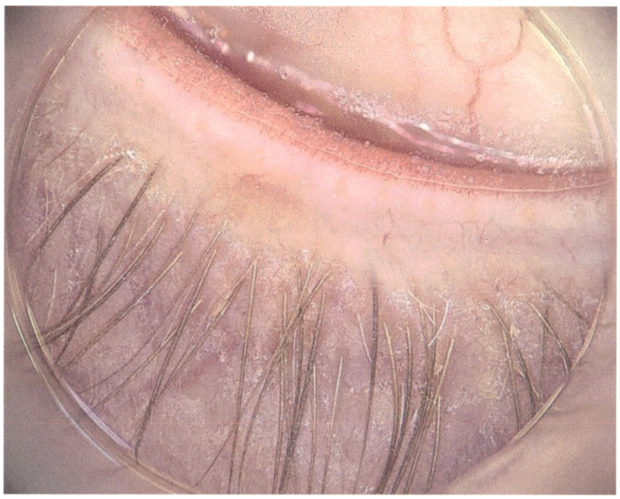

Figure 5.
A subtle junctional nevus close with a line of Meibomian glands. Courtesy of Pawel Pietkiewicz MD, PhD.

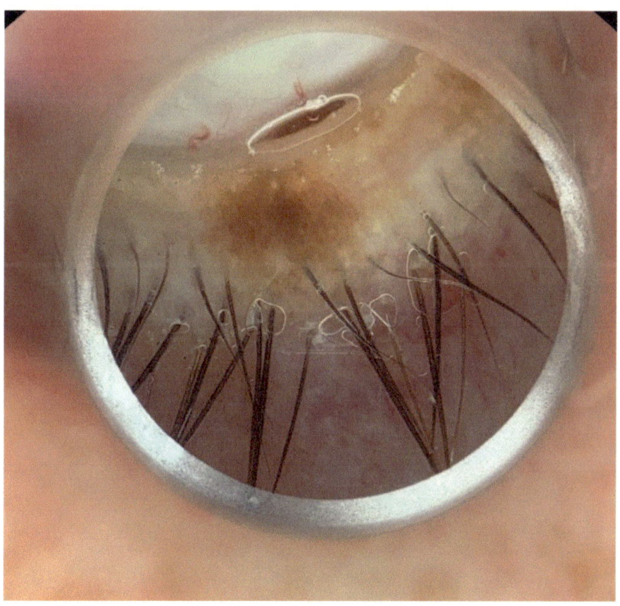

Figure 6.
A junctional nevus of the eyelid margin.

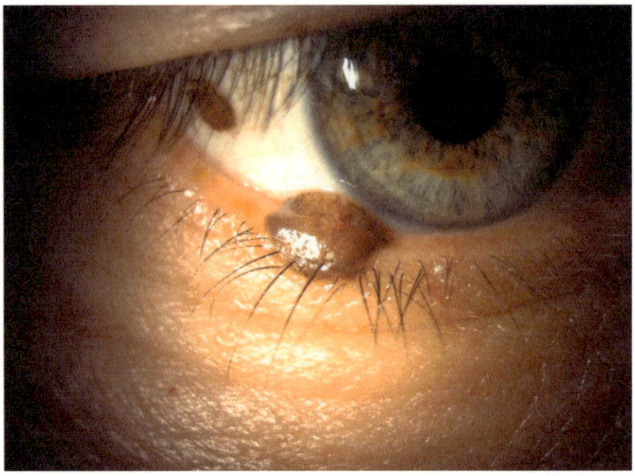

Figure 7.
Compound nevus of the eyelid margin with a junctional nevus of the conjunctiva.

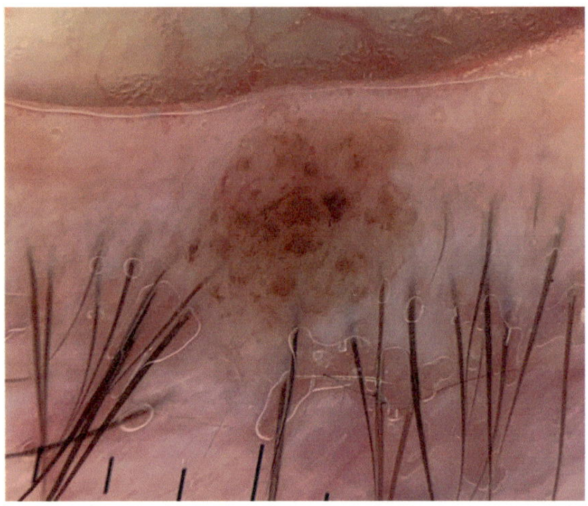

Figure 8.
Intradermal nevus of the eyelid margin – So called Miescher's nevus.

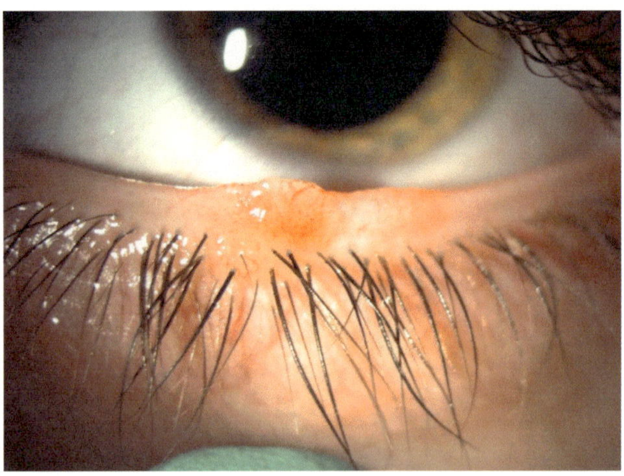

Figure 9.
An achromic intradermal nevus of the eyelid margin.

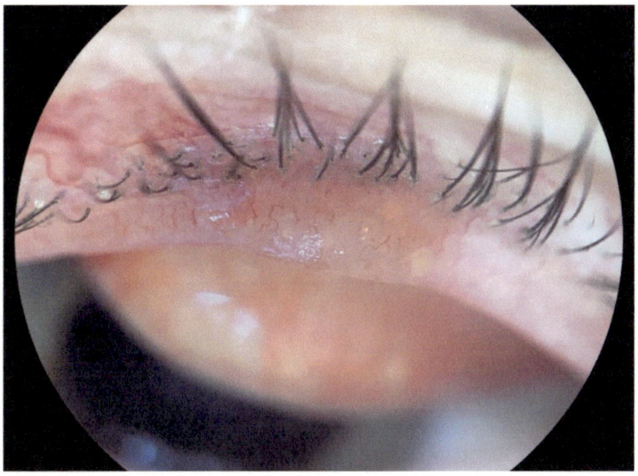

Figure 10.
An achromic intradermal nevus of the upper eyelid.

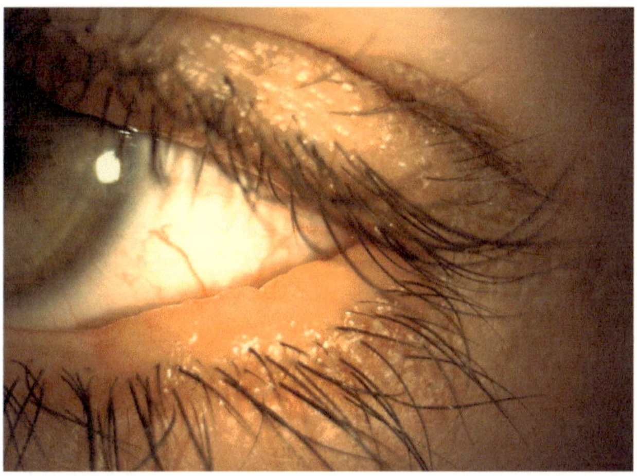

Figure 11.
An achromic kissing nevus of the upper and lower eyelid.

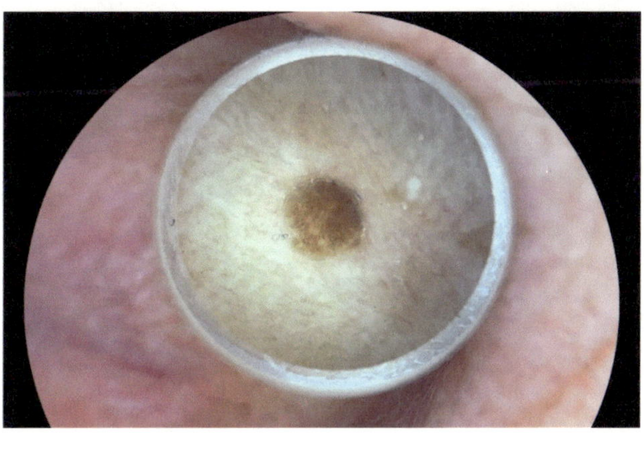

Figure 12.
An intradermal nevus as seen in dermatoscope.

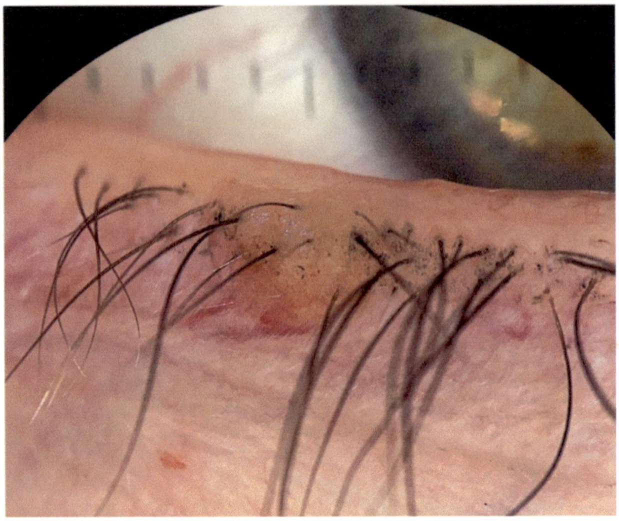

Figure 13.
An intradermal nevus of the eyelid margin.

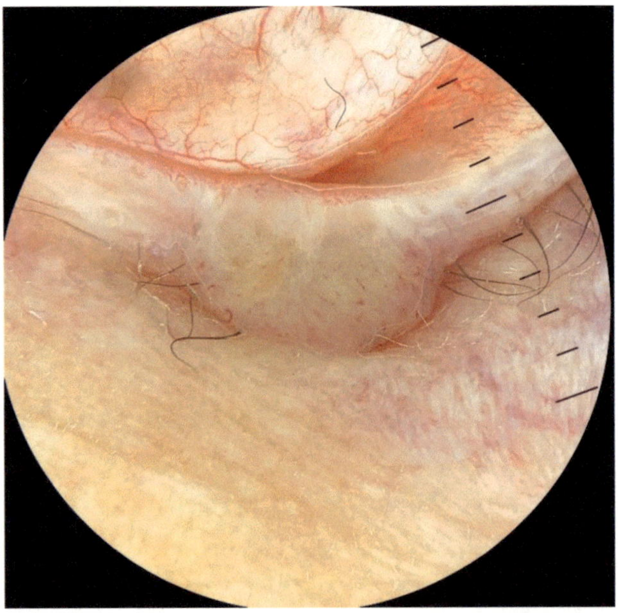

Figure 14.
A hypochromic intradermal nevus of the eyelid margin initially referenced as basal cell carcinoma.

pigmentation and brown globules are on the other hand more frequent in a nevi. Basal cell carcinoma has a more shiny and smooth surface, deprived of hair, whereas dermal nevus is more papilomatous with visible skin markings and hair follicles (**Figures 5–14**) [10].

3.8 Spitz and blue nevus

A Spitz and blue nevi are distinct types of melanocytic nevi. Their location in the eyelid area is extremely rare, and only a handful of cases have been described in the literature so far [11, 12].

4. Other benign lesions

4.1 Seborreheic keratosis

This benign skin lesion is a proliferation of basaloid cells. Although it is not composed of melanocytes, it may be pigmentary in appearance due to a transfer of melanin from them to the keratinocytes. It is usually a well-demarcated plaque or papilla [13]. Dermatoscopic features include fingerprinting or cerebrilike (brain-like) structures, comedo-like openings or pseudocomedones, moth-eaten borders, sharp demarcation and milia-like cysts, and centered looped vessels (**Figure 15**) [14].

4.2 Cystic lesions

The eyelid skin is rich with glandular tissue which may produce cystic lesions like epidermal inclusion cysts, hidrocystomas which appear when a gland duct is occluded. Those benign lesions may sometimes be misdiagnosed as malignant, especially when filled with blood or blood components that give them a pigmented appearance. The most typical dermatoscopic findings include the structureless pattern with cystic intradermal space filled with fluid and the presence of arborizing vessels (**Figures 16** and **17**) [15].

4.3 Malignant lesions

4.3.1 Melanoma

Melanoma of the eyelid region is sporadic, comprising less than 1% of all malignant eyelid lesion [16]. Due to the fact that the lower eyelid is much more exposed to ultraviolet light, melanoma appears much more commonly in this region compared to the upper eyelid [17]. It affects mainly patients with blond or red hair, pale skin, and the presence of multiple skin lesions, a tendency to burn and tan poorly, and a history of sunburn in childhood as well as artificial tanning before 25 years old.

The most common histological variants of melanoma in the eyelid area are lentigo maligna melanoma and superficial spreading melanoma [18, 19]. The most common dermatoscopic features include a higher number of dermatoscopic structures, and colors. The most prevalent pattern of melanoma in the face include gray

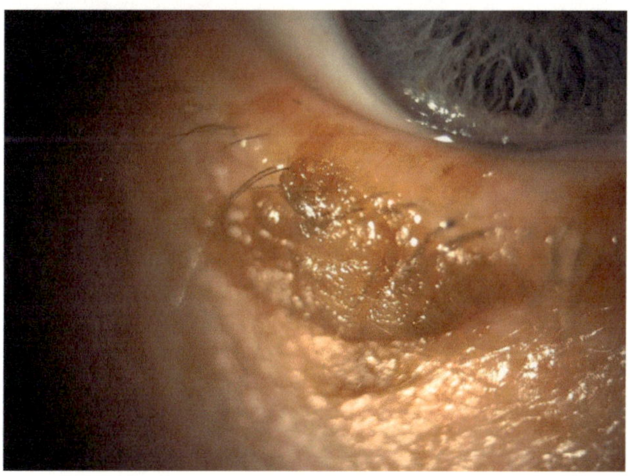

Figure 15.
Verruca seborrhoica.

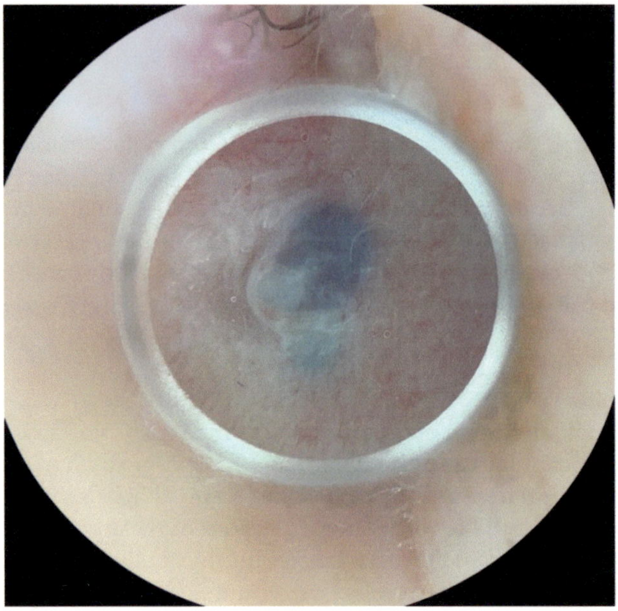

Figure 16.
Inclusion cyst filled with blood.

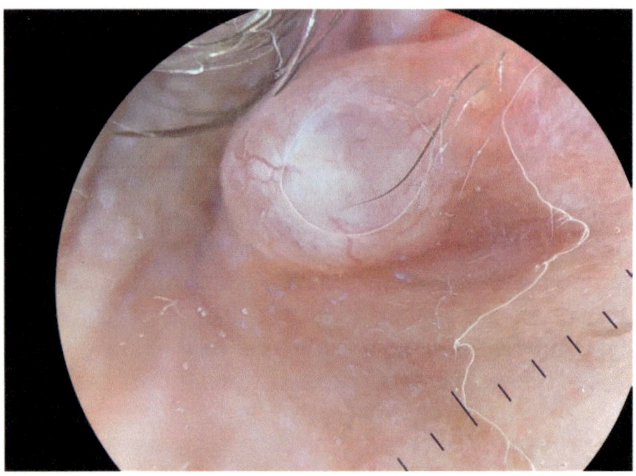

Figure 17.
Inclusion cyst of the eyelid margin.

color (homogenous areas, globules, dots, and circles), annular-granular pattern (dots aggregated around hair follicles), rhomboidal structures, and finally, obliterated hair follicles in invasive melanoma. Additional features include a shiny white line and a blue-whitish veil (**Figures 18** and **19**).

4.3.2 Basal cell carcinoma

Basal cell carcinoma (BCC) is the most common malignant skin lesion, accounting for 86% of all cutaneous malignancies. BCC is typically located in the lower eyelid or medial canthus. Clinically and histologically, the most common variants are the nodular, superficial, micronodular, morphiform, and pigmented. Pigmented BCC (pBCC) it is uncommon in light skin types, and more common in darker

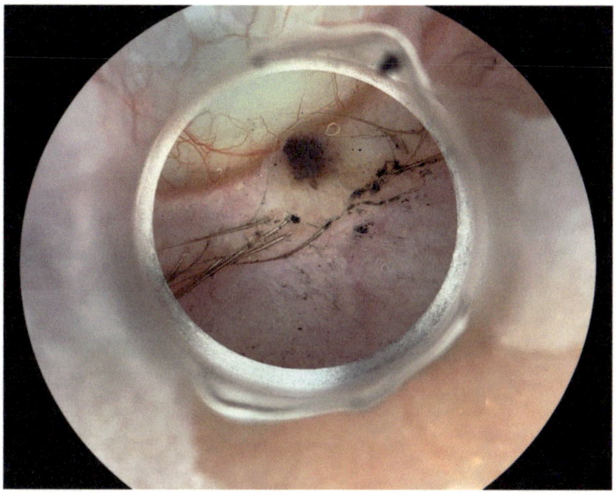

Figure 18.
A suspicious compound nevus of the eyelid margin.

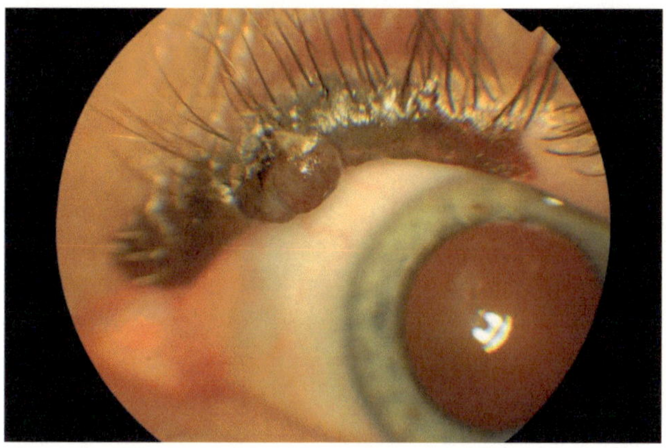

Figure 19.
Superficial spreading melanoma of the eyelid margin with a vertical nodular growth.

ones. The reason for the pigmented appearance of these lesions is that, that histologically they are composed of basaloid tumor cells intermingled with dendritic melanocytes. The melanocytes themselves usually do not demonstrate any atypical characteristics. No prognostic differences in pBCC are noted in comparison with clinically nonpigmented lesions [20]. Dermatoscopic features may vary. The most common dermatoscopic findings include arborizing vessels as well as mentioned above intense pink homogenous areas or yellow collor corresponding to ulceration. The vascular patterns may be different depending on the type of BCC. Nodular BCC usually presents with classical arborizing vessels while short telangiectasia suggests superficial BCC. Additional features may include leaf-like areas, spoke wheel-like areas, milia-like cysts, large ovoid nests, and target-like areas. Up to 10% of BCCs may contain pigmented structures like globules or dots [21–23]. Accurate dermatoscopic examination of the lesion borders may help plan surgical margins which may prove different than the ones observed surgically (**Figures 20** and **21**).

4.4 Conjunctival lesions

Infrequently, conjunctival lesions may also affect the eyelid margin. In the case of diffuse conjunctival infiltration, the involvement of eyelid skin should be

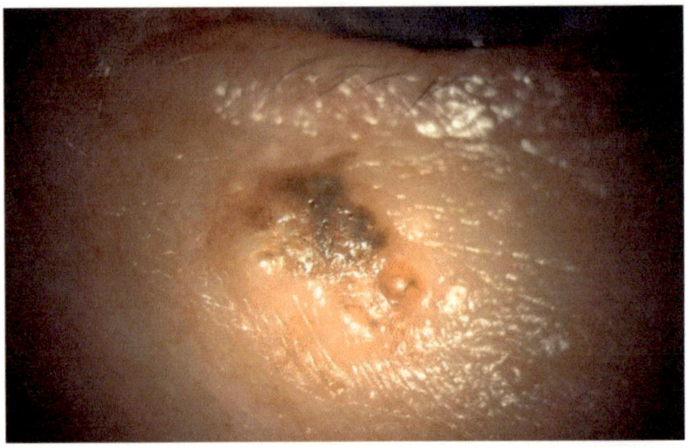

Figure 20.
Pigmentary basal cell carcinoma of the eyelid presenting shiny pearly-like surface.

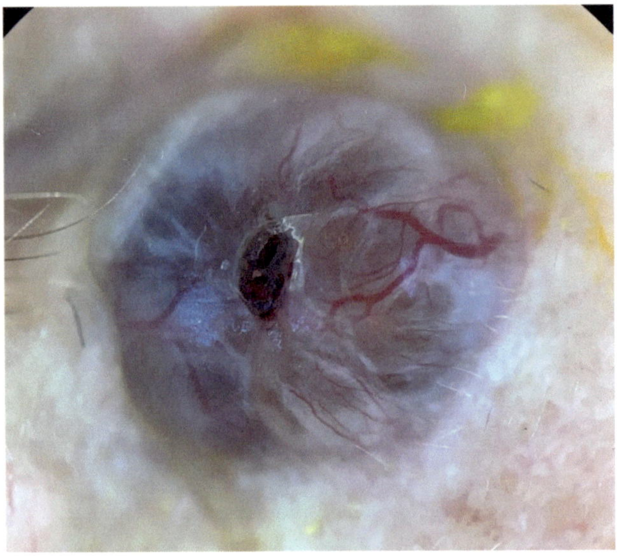

Figure 21.
Pigmentary basal cell carcinoma of the eyelid with ovoid nests, arborizing vesse, and central ulceration.

considered a poor prognostic factor. When noticing a melanocytic lesion of the eyelid margin, one should perform a precise assessment of the conjunctiva and conjunctival fornix, both the lower and the upper. Dermoscopic features of conjunctival melanoma were characterized as structureless areas, irregular dots, and a high prevalence of gray coloration [15]. Authors suggest that typical dermatoscopic features of skin melanoma may be also present in conjunctival melanoma such as atypical pigment network, irregular dots, and globules, regression structures, as well as blue-white veil (**Figure 22**) [24].

5. Lacrimal caruncle

While not specifically part of the eyelid region, the caruncle remains an interesting aspect. Although it may be confused with conjunctival tissue due to its proximity, it is, in fact, a skin fold covered with sebaceous and sweat glands located in the medial canthus of the eye. Due to its nature, although infrequently, it may be a point of origin for various skin lesions, mainly nevi or papillomas (**Figure 23**) [15, 25].

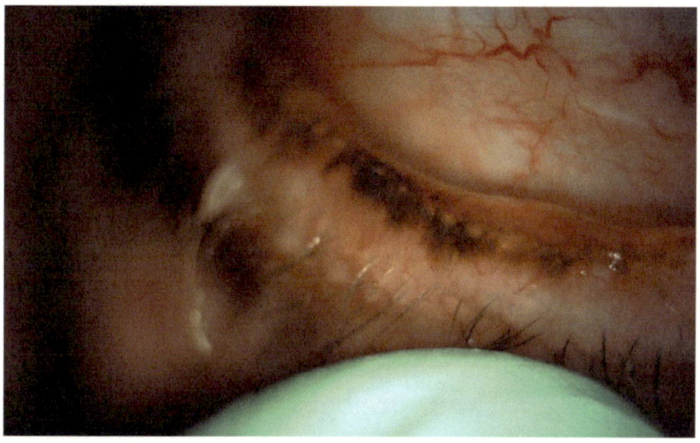

Figure 22.
Melanoma in situ of the conjunctiva, affecting the eyelid margin presenting black-brown-gray homogeneous area sparing hair follicle openings.

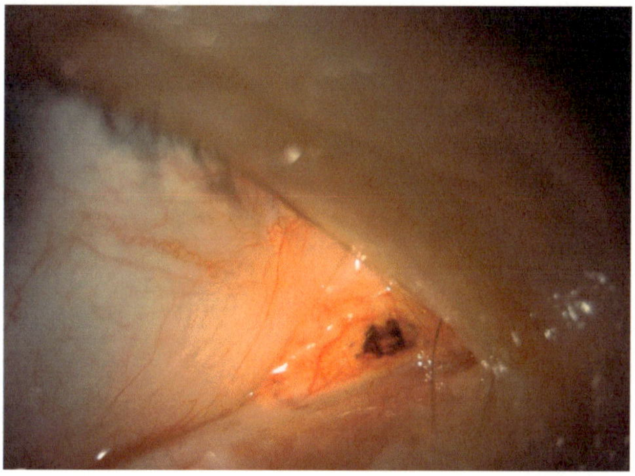

Figure 23.
Junctional nevus of the caruncle.

6. Approach to pigmented eyelid lesions

Because of the distinct anatomy of the eyelid, pigmented lesions of this area require a specific approach. Due to the eyelid being a very important cosmetic feature of the face, some patients pay special attention to lesions appearing in this region. Benign pigmented lesions may be removed by an ophthalmologist or an oculoplastic surgeon using surgery or other destructive methods such as cryotherapy or laser treatment after a careful dermatoscopic examination. Suspicious lesions require an incisional or excisional biopsy to determine their nature. Incisional biopsy should be chosen for large lesions, while small may undergo excisional biopsy.

Basal cell carcinoma with its pigmented variant may require Mohs micrographic surgery to safely assess its margins with the least healthy tissue traumatization.

General guidelines for the management of melanoma located in different areas of the body, where wide surgical excision is performed with margins according to the Breslow scale are not perfectly suitable for eyelid skin. It is caused by the specific anatomy of skin in this region and by the proximity of critical structures and difficulties with reconstructive surgery of large eyelid defects. Because of that, most surgeons suggest 3–5 mm surgical margins, however, this issue remains controversial, as some authors use up to 10 mm of safe surgical margin [17, 18, 26]. Long-term observations suggest a high rate of recurrence in the area of the head and neck.

Diffuse melanoma of the conjunctiva with the involvement of the eyelid region may require orbital exenteration which includes removal of the eyelids, the eyeball, and all surrounding tissues and remains a very traumatizing surgical procedure.

7. Conclusion

Because of the distinct anatomy of the eyelid, pigmentary lesions of this area require a specific, multidisciplinary approach including a dermatologist, ophthalmologist, oculoplastic surgeon, and oncologist.

Acknowledgements

All photographs presented in this chapter, unless stated otherwise, have been captured in Ocular Oncology Service, Department of Ophthalmology, Poznan University of Medical Sciences.

Conflict of interest

The authors declare no conflict of interest.

Author details

Wojciech Adamski[1] and Kinga Adamska[2]*

1 Department of Ophthalmology, Poznan University of Medical Sciences, Poznan, Poland

2 Psoriasis and Dermatology Modern Therapy Department, Poznan University of Medical Sciences, Poznan, Poland

*Address all correspondence to: kingabyczkowska@gmail.com

References

[1] Pratchyapruit W, Kikuchi K, Gritiyarangasan P, Aiba S, Tagami H. Functional analyses of the eyelid skin constituting the most soft and smooth area on the face: contribution of its remarkably large superficial corneocytes to effective water-holding capacity of the stratum corneum. Skin Research and Technology. 2007;**13**(2):169-175

[2] Font RL. Ophthalmic Pathology. In: An Atlas and Textbook. 3rd ed. Philadelphia: WB Saunders; 1996. Eyelids and lacrimal drainage system. pp. 2229-2232

[3] Ghias A, Asghar A, Ahmad TJ. Patterns of dermoscopy in common pigmented skin lesions. Journal of Pakistan Association of Dermatologists. 2017;**27**:346-352

[4] Jabłońska S, Majewski S. Choroby skóry i choroby przenoszone drogą płciową. Warszawa: Wydawnictwo Lekarskie PZWL; 2006

[5] Lodish MB, Stratakis CA. The differential diagnosis of familial lentiginosis syndromes. Familial Cancer. 2011;**10**(3):481-490

[6] McDonnell PJ, Mayou BJ. Congenital divided naevus of the eyelids. British Journal of Ophthalmology. 1988;**72**(3): 198-201

[7] Ritz M, Corrigan B. Congenital Melanocytic Nevi of the Eyelids and Periorbital Region. Plastic and Reconstructive Surgery. 2010;**125**(5): 1568-1569

[8] Swann PG, Kwong E. The naevus of Ota. Clinical and Experimental Optometry. 2010;**93**(4):264-267

[9] Hori Y, Kawashima M, Oohara K, Kukita A. Acquired, bilateral nevus of Ota-like macules. Journal of the American Academy of Dermatology. 1984;**10**(6):961-964

[10] Williams NM, Navarrete-Dechent C, Marghoob AA, Abarzua-Araya Á, Salerni G, Jaimes N. Differentiating basal cell carcinoma from intradermal nevi along the eyelid margin with dermoscopy: A case series. Journal of the American Academy of Dermatology. 2021;**84**(1):173-175

[11] Kirzhner M, Jakobiec FA, Kim N. Focal blue nevus of the eyelid margin (Mucocutaneous junction): A report of a unique case with a review of the literature. Ophthalmic Plastic & Reconstructive Surgery. 2011;**27**(5): 338-342

[12] Shields PW, Jakobiec FA, Stagner AM, Yoon MK. Spitz nevus arising in the eyelid of a teenager. Survey of Ophthalmology. 2016;**61**(2):228-235

[13] Deprez M, Uffer S. Clinico-pathological features of eyelid skin tumors. A retrospective study of 5504 cases and review of literature. The American Journal of Dermatopathology. 2009;**31**(3):256-262

[14] Cinotti E, La Rocca A, Labeille B, Grivet D, Lambert V, Kaspi M, et al. Dermoscopy for the diagnosis of eyelid margin tumours. The British Journal of Dermatology. 2019;**181**(2):397-398

[15] Kozubowska K, Sławińska M, Sobjanek M. The role of dermoscopy in diagnostics of dermatological conditions of the eyelid, eyelashes, and conjunctiva– A literature review. International Journal of Dermatology. 2021;**60**(8): 915-924

[16] Pe'er J, Folberg R. Eyelid tumors: Cutaneous melanoma. In: Pe'er J, Singh AD, editors. Clinical Ophthalmic Oncology: Eyelid and Conjunctival Tumors. 2nd ed. Berlin: Springer; 2014. pp. 63-68 Ch. 7

[17] Harish V, Bond JS, Scolyer RA, Haydu LE, Saw RPM, Quinn MJ, et al.

Margins of excision and prognostic factors for cutaneous eyelid melanomas. Journal of Plastic, Reconstructive & Aesthetic Surgery. 2013;**66**(8):1066-1073

[18] Chan FM, O'Donnell BA, Whitehead K, Ryman W, Sullivan TJ. Treatment and outcomes of malignant melanoma of the eyelid. Ophthalmology. 2007;**114**(1):187-192

[19] Pietkiewicz P. Lentiginous melanoma – should we change the paradigm? Journal of the European Academy of Dermatology and Venereology. 2021;**35**(6):1246-1247

[20] Cameron MC, Lee E, Hibler BP, Barker CA, Mori S, Cordova M, et al. Basal cell carcinoma: Epidemiology; pathophysiology; clinical and histological subtypes; and disease associations. Journal of the American Academy of Dermatology. 2019;**80**(2):303-317

[21] Reiter O, Mimouni I, Gdalevich M, et al. The diagnostic accuracy of dermoscopy for basal cell carcinoma: A systematic review and meta-analysis. Journal of the American Academy of Dermatology. 2019;**80**:1380

[22] Haws AL, Rojano R, Tahan SR, Phung TL. Accuracy of biopsy sampling for subtyping basal cell carcinoma. Journal of the American Academy of Dermatology. 2012;**66**:106

[23] Papageorgiou C, Apalla Z, Variaah G, et al. Accuracy of dermoscopic criteria for the differentiation between superficial basal cell carcinoma and Bowen's disease. Journal of the European Academy of Dermatology and Venereology. 2018;**32**:1914-1919

[24] Li K, Xin L. Palpebral conjunctiva melanoma with dermoscopic and clinicopathological characteristics. Journal of the American Academy of Dermatology. 2014;**71**(2):e35-e37

[25] Santos A, Gómez-Leal A. Lesions of the Lacrimal Caruncle. Ophthalmology. 1994;**101**(5):943-949

[26] Collgros H, Rodriguez-Lomba E, Regio Pereira A, Lo SN, Scolyer RA, Guitera P. Lentiginous melanoma (lentigo maligna and lentigo maligna melanoma) in Australia: Clinicopathological characteristics, management and recurrence rates after 10-year follow-up at a tertiary centre. Journal of the European Academy of Dermatology and Venereology. 2021;**35**(6):1315-1322

Section 5

Miscellaneous

Chapter 6

Dermatoscopic Findings in Palmoplantar Dermatoses

Tubanur Çetinarslan, Ece Gökyayla and Aylin Türel Ermertcan

Abstract

Dermatoscopy is a useful, non-invasive method in the diagnosis of various dermatological diseases. Dermatoscopy of non-pigmented skin lesions shows additional morphologic features, such as cutaneous vascular pattern, scale color and scale distribution pattern, and background color. Dermatoscopy can be useful tool in differential diagnosis in palmoplantar dermatoses. The most specific dermatoscopic features of hand eczema include yellowish-orange globules, yellowish scales and yellowish crusts. Light red background color, regular vascular distribution pattern, dotted vessels and white scale color have been reported in previous studies as dermatoscopic features of palmoplantar psoriasis. Dotted vessels can be seen in various dermatoses, such as psoriasis, eczema, lichen planus, porokeratosis and keratodermas. The distribution pattern and color of the scales are also important in the differential diagnosis of palmoplantar dermatoses. Previous studies have shown that scales are mainly localized in skin furrows in patients with tinea manum. Patchy distributed, homogeneous, structureless, orange areas were reported in palmar keratoderma due to pityriasis rubra pilaris. Amber scales, white-to-pinkish background; sparse whitish scales were reported in palmar keratoderma due to mycosis fungoides. Dermatoscopical findings of palmoplantar area can help in the differential diagnosis of various dermatoses.

Keywords: dermatoscopy, palmoplantar, eczema, psoriasis, tinea manuum

1. Introduction

Dermatoscopy is a useful, non-invasive and cost-effective diagnostic tool for benign and malignant skin tumors; it is also important in the clinical diagnosis of pigmentary disorders, hair-nail disorders, inflammatory and infectious diseases [1].

Palmoplantar dermatoses include a wide range of skin conditions. Dermatological diseases involving palmoplantar region are a common question when consulted in dermatological practice. The correct diagnosis is often easy on the basis of typical clinical characteristics, but could be difficult when several entities occur at the same time or overlap.

Many dermatological diseases can involve palmoplantar region; such as inflammatory dermatoses, infections and palmoplantar keratodermas (PPKs). In particular, differential diagnosis of inflammatory dermatoses such as eczema, psoriasis, pityriasis rubra pilaris (PRP), lichen planus may be more difficult in patients with isolated involvement of the palmoplantar region.

2. Dermatoscopic findings in palmoplantar dermatoses

2.1 Inflammatory dermatoses

Dermatoscopy has been shown to be a useful supportive tool to assist the diagnosis of inflammatory skin diseases [2–10].

In this section, dermatoscopical findings in inflammatory dermatoses localized in the palmoplantar region will be discussed.

2.1.1 Psoriasis vulgaris

Psoriasis is a common skin disorder that can affect people of all ages. Chronic plaque psoriasis (psoriasis vulgaris) is the most common form of the disease, and accounts for about 90% of cases [11]. Psoriasis can affect any skin site. Palmoplantar plaque psoriasis is a manifestation of plaque psoriasis which affects the palms and soles [12]. It could present as isolated palmoplantar involvement or may be associated with generalized psoriasis vulgaris [13, 14].

There are few studies in the literature regarding the use of dermatoscopy in palmoplantar psoriasis [2–4]. Dermatoscopy of palmoplantar plaque psoriasis shows a characteristic pattern consisting of diffuse white scales and symmetrically, regularly distributed dotted vessels on a light or dull red background [1–6]. It has been reported that the scale distribution pattern is rarely central or patchy [2, 5].

Although dotted vessels are a hallmark of trunk and extremity plaque psoriasis [6], as well as palmoplantar involvement [2], it should be remarked that this finding is not specific for psoriasis vulgaris. It could also be seen in eczema [2, 3], Bowen's disease [7], lichen nitidus [8], lichen simplex chronicus [15] and PRP [5, 9, 16]. Based on these findings, it can be suggested that dotted vessels may not be useful to distinguish psoriasis from other dermatoses, but the vascular distribution pattern may be beneficial in the differential diagnosis [2, 3, 17, 18].

Regular dotted vessels are the most common vascular distribution pattern in palmoplantar psoriasis [2, 3, 18]. Yu et al. found that beaded distributed dotted vessels along the sulci cutis is important new finding in psoriasis. It has been suggested that this finding, which is not seen in palmoplantar eczema, may be useful in differential diagnosis [4]. **Figure 1a** shows clinical view of palmar psoriasis vulgaris and **Figure 1b** shows regular dotted vessels on light red background.

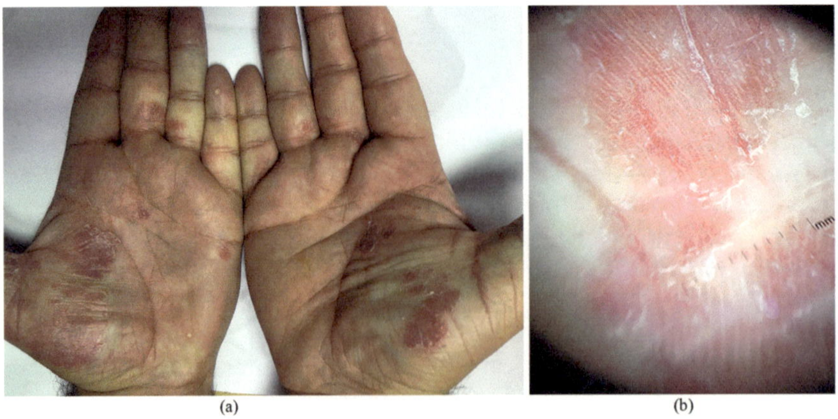

(a) (b)

Figure 1.
(a) Palmar psoriasis vulgaris. (b) Regular dotted vessels on a light red background.

Vazquez-Lopez et al. described the vascular pattern that they specifically named "red globular rings" in plaque psoriasis lesions [19]. Lacarrubba et al. reported this pattern is a less common, but specific vascular pattern in plaque psoriasis lesions [20]. We showed red globular ring vessels in psoriasis also in palmoplantar lesions. Rarely, other vessel types have been reported in palmoplantar region [2].

Micali et al. showed dilated/tortuous "bushy" capillaries in all of the patients with palmar and/or plantar psoriasis by using videodermatoscopy. On the other hand, this pattern was not detected in patients with palmar and/or plantar eczema. Normal capillary pattern or dilated capillaries without tortuous or "bushy" appearance were showed in eczema [21].

The background color of the lesion, scale color and scale distribution pattern are useful findings to differentiate inflammatory dermatoses [2–10, 22].

Diffuse white scale is the most common scale distribution pattern in both the body and palmoplantar psoriasis lesions. The presence of diffuse white scales in psoriasis could explain with the dry and hyperkeratotic nature of plaque psoriasis [1, 15, 23]. Central and peripheral scale distribution patterns are very rare in psoriasis [2]. **Figure 2a** shows clinical view of palmar psoriasis and **Figure 1b** shows diffuse white scales along with the skin furrows. **Figure 3a** shows diffuse white scales in palmar plaque psoriasis.

It is recommended to examine the vascular structures after the scale is removed because of difficulty to show the vascular structures in palmoplantar region due to the presence of hyperkeratosis [3, 6, 24, 25]. In addition, it is suggested to use a fluid interface to reduce the scaling [6].

Lallas et al. examined the background color of the lesions in patients with plaque psoriasis, eczema, pityriasis rosea and lichen planus affecting the trunk and /or upper or lower extremities. They found that the most common background color was light red in psoriasis and, white versus yellow scales along with regular versus patchy distribution of dotted vessels may represent a valuable clue in the differential diagnosis of plaque psoriasis and nummular eczema [22]. Similarly, we found that light red is the most common background color in patients with palmoplantar psoriasis [2].

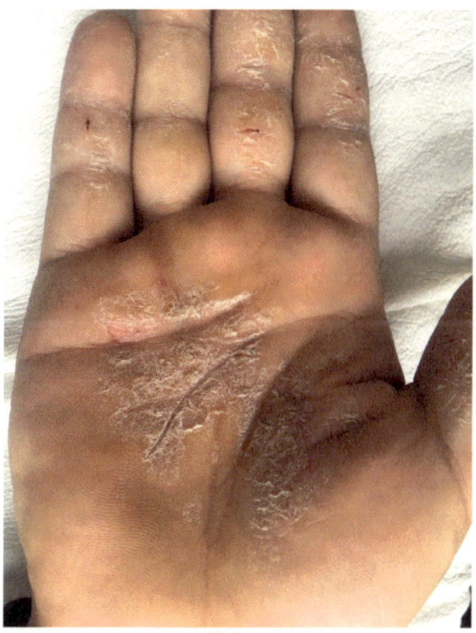

(a)

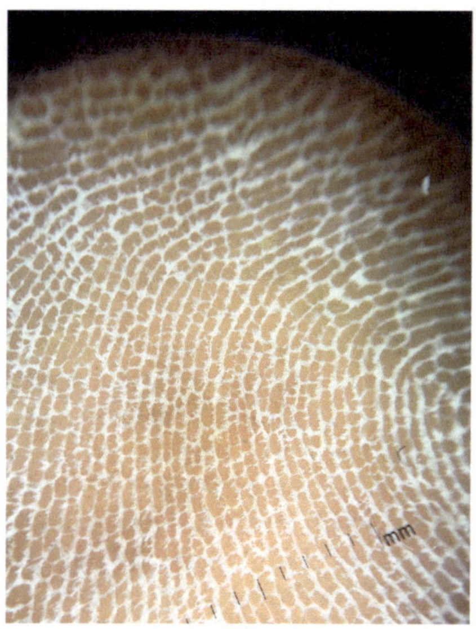

(b)

Figure 2.
(a) Palmar psoriasis vulgaris. (b) Diffuse white scales along with the skin furrows.

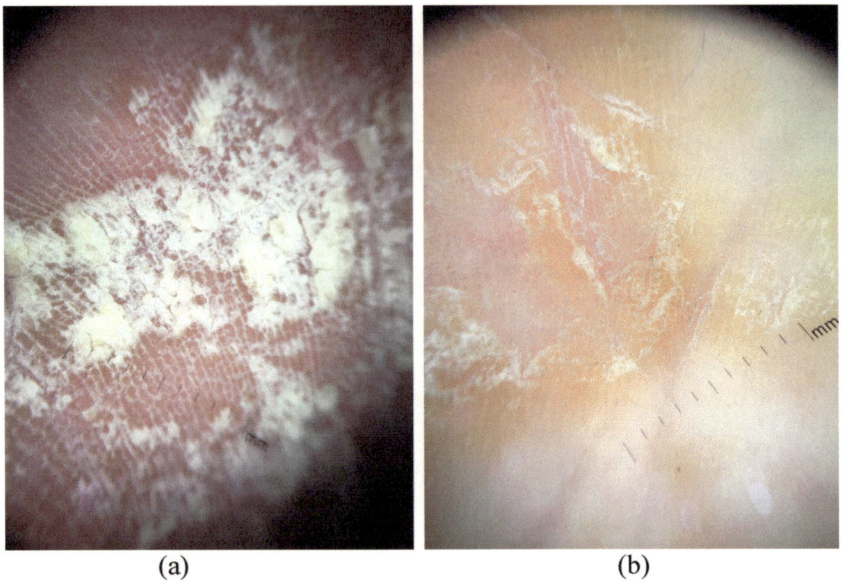

Figure 3.
(a) Diffuse white scales in palmar psoriasis. (b) Yellowish background and patchy yellow scales in eczema.

Specific clues can also be used in the differential diagnosis of inflammatory dermatoses. Palmar papular psoriasis can be differentiated from porokeratosis, with the absence of peripheral annular whitish keratotic track [26], and lichen planus, which is characterized by the detection of Wickham striae [26, 27].

In a recent study, Yu et al. investigated 26 patients with palmoplantar psoriasis and 31 patients with palmoplantar eczema. The most common dermatoscopic appearance of psoriasis was a red background, white scales, and dotted/globular/hairpin type vessels in a regular arrangement, while the presence of pink background, yellow scales, and atypical blood vessels in an irregular arrangement were observed in eczema. The most specific dermatoscopical finding in psoriasis was hairpin type vessels (100%), and followed by regular arrangement of blood vessels (93.55%), red background color (87.1%), dotted or globular vessels (77.42%), and white scales (54.84%). They suggested that regular arrangement of vessels was the most valuable finding for the diagnosis of palmoplantar psoriasis and they reported that dotted vessels in beaded distribution pattern along the sulci cutis that cannot always be shown was very specific for psoriasis. They suggested that the most characteristic dermatoscopical finding of psoriasis is the regular distributed hairpin/dots/globular vessels. It is assumed that the appearance of these vascular structures changes according to the position of the dermatoscope. When dermatoscope is perpendicular to dilated capillaries dotted/globular type vessels could be seen, ring/hairpin type vessels could be seen when viewed with angle. Yu et al. showed hairpin type vessels in 34.6% of PP patients. However, they suggested that hairpin type vessels show a high diagnostic specificity for psoriasis. They also reported that, unlike in other studies [2, 3], the color of the scales was not significant in the differential diagnosis of eczema and psoriasis in the palmoplantar region [4].

Lallas et al. investigated 22 palmoplantar psoriasis lesions (14 on palms and 8 on soles) under dermatoscopy. They showed diffuse white scales and regular dotted vessels. Dotted vessels were seen in 90% of lesions, this ratio was the lowest compared to other body parts. They explained this finding by the thickness of the epidermis of palmoplantar region, which possibly impedes the visualization. They showed white scales in all palmoplantar lesions [6].

We examined dermatoscopic findings of 90 patients, 35 palmoplantar pustular psoriasis and 55 palmoplantar hyperkeratotic eczema. Similar to other studies, we showed red background color, regular vascular distribution pattern, red globular ring vessels and white scale color in psoriasis in our study [2].

2.1.2 Pustular psoriasis

Palmoplantar pustular psoriasis (PPP) is a chronic immune-mediated skin disease that mainly affects women in the fourth to seventh decade of life. It is a debilitating disease of the palms and/or soles and show high resistance to treatment [28]; in addition has a high impact on health-related life quality [29]. PPP is characterized by eruptive, sterile intraepidermal pustules on the palms and soles, with psoriasis vulgaris-like erythematous and desquamating lesions [14].

Pustular psoriasis shows yellow globules correspond to non-follicular superficial pustules; and regularly distributed dotted vessels correspond to papillary dermal vessels dilatation. In addition, white or yellow scales or crusts may also occur [5, 10, 15, 30].

Although pustules are not visible on clinical examination, yellow globules may be seen with dermatoscopy even at initial stages [30–32].

Palmoplantar pustulosis, or pustulosis palmaris et plantaris, is a chronic inflammatory and recurrent skin disease with clinical findings of erythema, scales and pustules on the palms and soles. In the advanced stage, the lesions consist of numerous pustules on an erythematous-squamous base [33]. To the our knowledge, there is no previous report about dermatoscopical findings in palmoplantar pustulosis. We showed white scales, yellow globules and regular dotted vessels similar to palmoplantar pustular psoriasis. **Figure 4a** shows clinical view of palmoplantar pustulosis and **Figure 4b** shows yellow globules, white scales and regular dotted vessels.

2.2 Eczema

Chronic hand eczema (CHE) clinically presents with sharply demarcated areas of thick scaling or hyperkeratosis on the proximal or middle aspect of the palms [34]. Eczematous dermatitis shows some differences according to the disease stage. Acute exudative lesions represent yellow scales/crusts and chronic lesions demonstrate patched distributed dotted vessels with scaling [15, 22, 35].

The characteristic dermatoscopic findings of CHE include yellowish scales, brownish-orange dots/globules, and yellowish-orange crusts [3, 5]. **Figure 3b** shows yellowish background and patchy yellow scales in eczema.

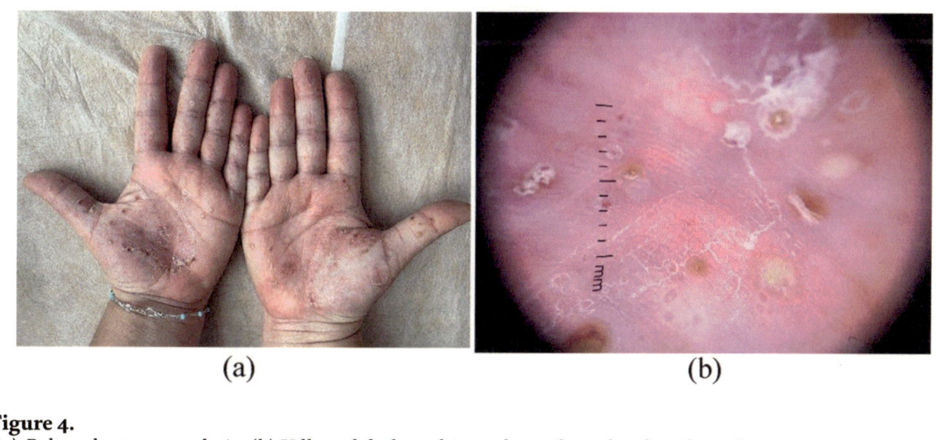

(a) (b)

Figure 4.
(a) Palmoplantar pustulosis. (b) Yellow globules, white scales and regular dotted vessels.

Patchy dotted vessels with yellow scales are indicative of eczema in body and extremity lesions [22]. Errichetti et al. suggested that dermatoscopic features of CHE is similar to eczematous dermatitis localized on other sites. Dermatoscopic features of CHE includes yellowish scaling with or without white scales, yellowish crusts and focal dotted vessels [1, 15, 23]. Similar to previous studies [18, 22], patchy vascular distribution pattern and dotted vessels have also been demonstrated in the palmoplantar region of eczema patients [2, 3]. Glomerular, linear and hairpin vessels have been rarely reported in CHE [2, 3].

Errichetti et al. reported dermatoscopic findings of 10 patients with palmar psoriasis and 11 patients with CHE. Yellowish scales, brownish-orange dots/globules and yellowish-orange crusts have been shown in CHE. It was suggested that the presence of brownish-orange dots/globules corresponds to tiny spongiotic vesicles. Palmoplantar spongiotic vesicles have a higher resistance to rupture compared with other areas because of the increased thickness of the keratin layer at these sites [3]. Similarly, we showed yellow-orange crusts, patchy vascular distribution pattern, brownish-orange globules, yellow scale color and dull red background color in CHE in our study [2]. Yu et al. found that brown-orange-yellow dots are significant for the diagnosis of palmoplantar eczema [4]. Yellowish scales, brownish orange dots/globules and yellowish-orange crusts show the spongiotic nature of CHE [1, 3].

Figure 5a shows clinical view of dyshidrotic eczema and **Figure 5b** shows yellowish background, brownish-orange globules and yellow scales in dyshidrotic eczema.

We also observed globule structures with pale center and dark peripheral rim only in patients with CHE, which was thought due to spongiosis progressing to vesicle formation that suggesting eczema. Dark peripheral rim may be associated with hyperkeratotic foci around vesicles [2]. **Figure 6a** shows globule structures with pale center and dark peripheral rim in CHE. **Figure 6b** shows yellowish background, brownish-orange globules and yellow scales in CHE.

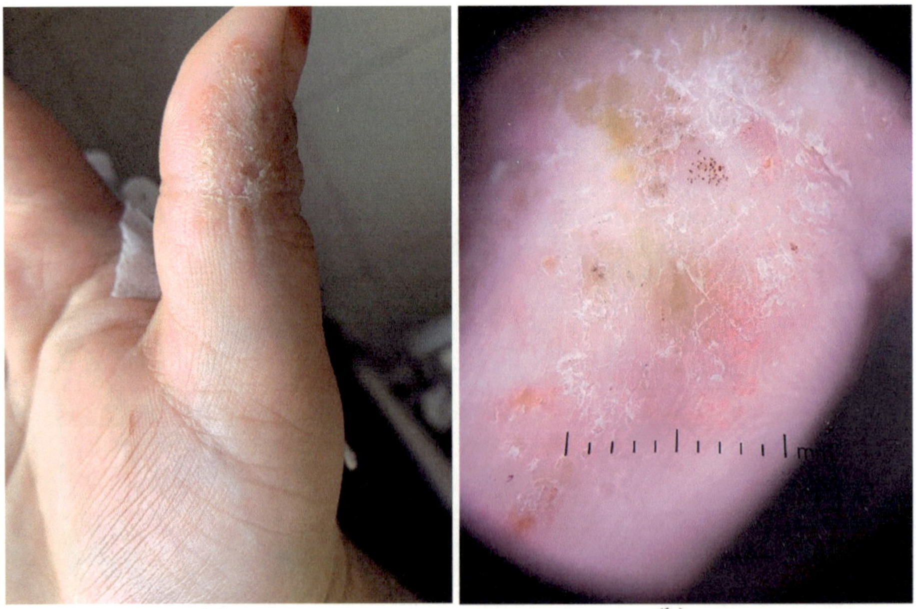

(a) (b)

Figure 5.
(a) Dyshidrotic eczema. (b) Yellowish background, brownish-orange globules and yellow scales in dyshidrotic eczema.

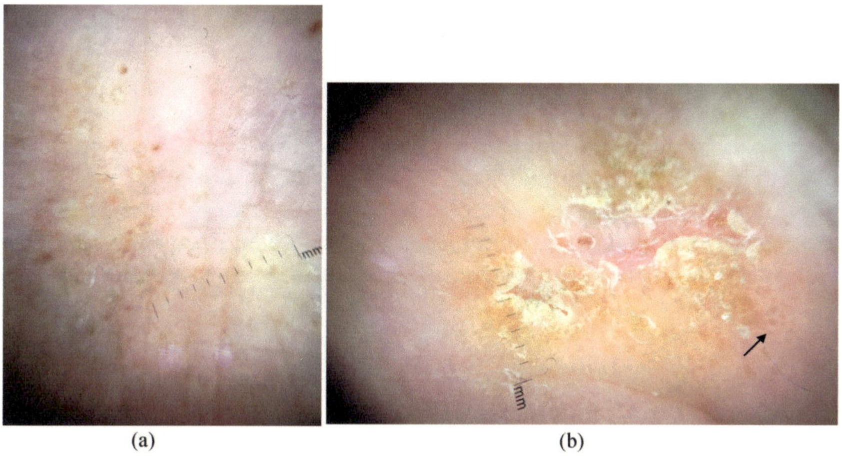

Figure 6.
(a) Globule structures with pale center and dark peripheral rim in chronic hand eczema. (b) Yellowish background, brownish-orange globules and yellow scales in chronic hand eczema.

Errichetti et al. noticed a higher prevalence of scaling than vessels compared to other studies. This difference could be explained by the use of an interface fluid in the previous studies which improved the visualization of the vessels [6].

It has been suggested that the color of scales (white vs. yellow) is the most useful clue for distinguishing psoriasis and eczematous dermatitis in body localizations [1, 15, 23]. In previous studies, yellow is the main scale color in palmoplantar eczema [2, 3]. The histopathological reason for this color is irregular hyperplasia of the spinous layer, spongiotic edema, and serous exudation of the cuticle layer [4].

Unlike other studies, Yu et al. suggested that scale color in palmoplantar psoriasis is similar to eczema because of the topical drug usage and the presence of a thicker corneous layer. They also showed atypical vessels and dark red stasis around cracks in palmoplantar eczema. This finding could be explained by itch-provoked excoriations [4]. **Figure 4a** shows globule structures with pale center and dark peripheral rim in chronic hand eczema and **Figure 4b** shows yellowish background, brownish-orange globules and yellow scales in CHE.

2.3 Keratodermas

Palmoplantar keratodermas (PPKs) are diverse group of disorders that are characterized by abnormal thickening of the skin on the palms and soles. PPKs may be divided into acquired and genetic types [36].

Acquired PPKs lesions have a wide range of clinical appearances: diffuse, focal, and punctate. There are many causes of acquired PPKs [37].

In this section, dermatoscopic findings of PPKs will be discussed. There are a few publications on dermatoscopy of PPKs in the literature.

2.3.1 Keratoderma due to pityriasis rubra pilaris

PRP is an inflammatory skin disease, and its most common presentation is characterized by follicular and palmoplantar hyperkeratosis and orange-red scaling plaques [38].

Papular lesions of classic PRP usually reveal round/oval yellowish areas surrounded by vessels of mixed morphology (i.e., linear and dotted) and often centered by central keratin plugs on body lesions [10, 15, 25, 39]. It has been suggested that orange-colored areas in PRP-related acquired keratoderma is compatible with the clinical finding of such a tint in PRP [25, 40, 41].

There is only one report in the literature reporting dermatoscopic findings in palmar keratoderma due to PRP. Errichetti et al. reported dermatoscopic findings in four palmar acquired keratoderma patients (1 psoriasis, 1 eczema, 1 PRP, 1 mycosis fungoides (MF)) in their study. They reported monomorphous aspect consisting of whitish scaling with patchy distributed, homogeneous, structureless, orange areas presenting with different sizes in palmar acquired keratoderma due to PRP. Non-specific dermatoscopic structures, including whitish scaling and reddish fissures could be seen [25].

2.3.2 Keratoderma due to mycosis fungoides

Mycosis fungoides (MF), the most common cutaneous T-cell lymphoma, typically presents with inflammatory erythematous patches or plaques in its early stage. There is only one publication in the literature reporting dermatoscopic findings in palmar acquired keratoderma due to MF. It has been observed relatively large, amber scales over a white-to-pinkish background; sparse whitish scales and several non-specific reddish fissures in palmar acquired keratoderma due to MF [25].

They concluded that the presence of large amber scales and a pale background in MF-related acquired keratoderma might be due to the marked/compact hyperkeratosis/acanthosis [25, 40, 42].

2.3.3 Aquagenic syringeal acrokeratoderma

Aquagenic syringeal acrokeratoderma (ASA) is a rare acquired condition characterized by translucent papules and plaques with apparent eccrine duct openings. The lesions appear only after a 2- to 4-minute exposure to water. ASA is more common on palmar surface, although the dorsal surfaces of the hands and plantar region could also be involved [43].

Fernández-Crehuet et al. investigated four patients with ASA and, observed the presence of well-defined yellowish globules not affecting dermatoglyphics in all of their patients. They suggested that these structures could be due to widening of the excretory ducts of eccrine sweat glands [44].

Sezer et al. found larger sweat duct pores compared with normal palmar region, reflecting the dilated and tortuous acrosyringium [45].

Lacarrubba et al. showed a hypertrophic stratum corneum with deepening of normal dermatoglyphics and a marked dilatation of eccrine ostia, both configuring a gruyere-like aspect in a 19-year-old woman with cystic fibrosis [46].

2.4 Lichen planus

Palmoplantar lichen planus (LP) is an uncommon localized variant of lichen planus [47].

Errichetti et al. reported that palmar LP is characterized by roundish yellowish areas often having peripheral projections that may create a star-like appearance; a purplish background is sometimes visible [5].

Wickham striae are typically white, they could also appear yellow on palmoplantar areas [5, 10, 15].

Figure 7a shows clinical view of palmoplantar LP. **Figure 7b** shows brownish areas and Wickham stria on a purplish background.

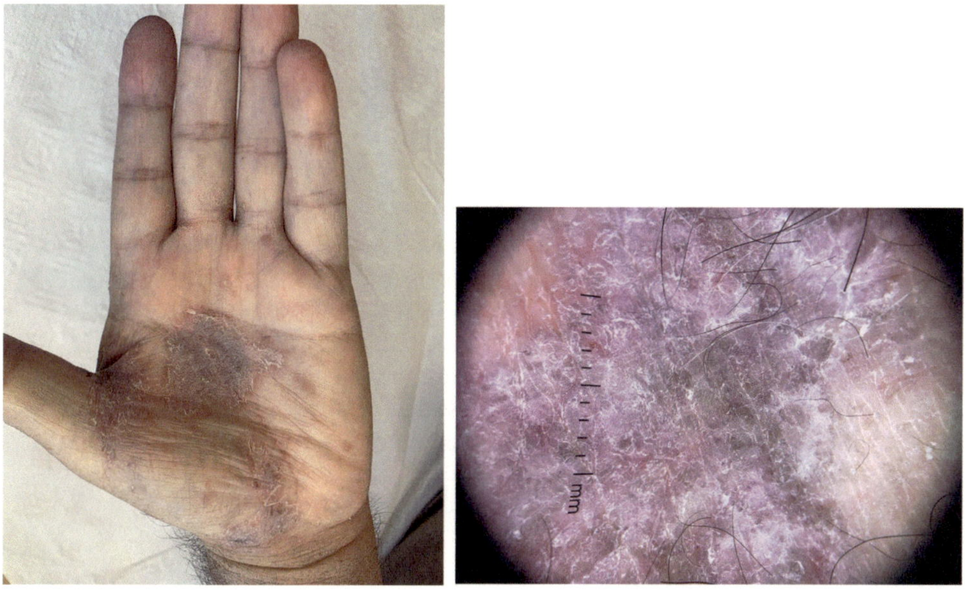

(a) (b)

Figure 7.
(a) Palmar lichen planus. (b) Brownish areas and Wickham stria on a purplish background.

2.5 Lichen nitidus

Lichen nitidus is a relatively uncommon chronic inflammatory disease which is presented with 1–2 mm, shiny, flat-topped, pale to skin-colored, clustered papules. The lesions mostly seen over the penis, lower abdomen, medial surface of the thighs, dorsal hands, forearms and buttocks [48]. It can be seen on palmoplantar region, nail and mucosa uncommonly [49].

Qian et al. reported well-defined depressions with fewer, thinner scales, surrounded with obvious ring-shaped, silvery-white scales on the palmoplantar sites. They suggested that the variation of pit patterns on palmoplantar area under dermatoscopy depends on epidermal hyperkeratosis, persistent mechanical stress, and thickness of stratum corneum. On the other hand, dermatoscopical findings of lichen nitidus on other localizations showed round, elevated, shiny and smooth surface without scales in their study [50].

3. Infectious diseases

Dermatoscopy is a helpful tool in the diagnosis of various infectious diseases. In this section, dermatoscopic findings reported on infectious diseases involving the palmoplantar region will be discussed.

3.1 Tinea manuum

Tinea manuum is a superficial mycosis of the palm, dorsum, or interdigital folds of one or both hands. It is usually caused by dermatophytes [41].

Errichetti et al. reported that whitish scaling mainly located in the furrows is specific for tinea manuum. They explained this finding with the localization of dermatophytes to proliferate in moist environment, such as palmar furrows [13].

Jakhar et al. also reported that dotted vessels only in the skin furrows is another dermatoscopic finding in tinea manuum. They explained this vascular finding with the reactionary vasodilatation of vessels in response to inflammatory process induced by dermatophytes [5, 51, 52].

3.2 Tinea nigra

Tinea nigra (TN) is a rare superficial cutaneous mycosis caused by Hortaea werneckii. Dermatoscopy is a fast and effective tool for the diagnostic suspicion of TN. Multiple light brown thin lines that cross forming a weave is characteristic dermatoscopic finding in TN [53]. Navarrete et al. also defined hyperchromic patch with a regular distribution of the pigmentation and the spicules on the edges [54]. Guarenti et al. examined an 11-year-old girl with TN and demonstrated a homogeneous nonmelanocytic pigmented pattern with spicules [55]. The pigmentation in TN does not follow the parallel ridges pattern described for melanomas [39]. However, there are some reported cases contrary to this information [56, 57].

3.3 Palmar syphiloderm

Syphilis is a chronic, systemic infection that mimics many dermatological diseases. Secondary syphilis is classically characterized by a copper- colored maculopapular rash with sharply delineated margins typically present on the palmar and plantar surfaces [13].

Errichetti et al. showed an orangish background and a thin, whitish, annular, scaling edge progressing in an outward direction and often surrounded by an erythematous halo in palmar syphiloderm [27].

It has been suggested that the presence of an orangish background corresponds to hemosiderin deposits in the dermis as a consequence of extravasation of erythrocytes, typical for secondary syphilitic lesions [5]. Palmar syphilis lesions may be confused with palmar papular psoriasis. Palmar papular psoriasis shows no orangish areas/background and, this has been emphasized as an important finding in differential diagnosis. The diffuse/regular distributed dotted vessels may be seen in both psoriasis and palmar syphiloderm, consequently it may not be useful in the differential diagnosis [58].

Tognetti et al. showed a circular, thin, scaling edge progressing in an outward direction and surrounded by an erythematous halo (the so-called Biett's collarette) as a diagnostic indicator, even in clinically non-scaling lesions in palmar syphiloderm [58]. Errichetti et al. reported thicker scaling ring and lacking of erythematous halo [3, 6, 25].

3.4 Pitted keratolysis

Pitted keratolysis is a bacterial infection of plantar region which caused by Gram-positive bacteria, especially *Corynebacterium spp* [59]. Hyperhidrosis, long standing occlusion and increased skin pH are predisposing factors. In an appropriate environment, bacteria proliferate and secrete keratin-degrading enzymes which are responsible for pitted appearance. Patients usually present with irritated, malodored, hyperhidrotic soles with small, multiple pits on them. Lockwood et al. identified dermatoscopy of pitted keratolysis in a case report as irregularly distributed pits with heterogeneously architecture pit walls [60].

3.5 Verruca plantaris

Verruca plantaris is a common human papilloma virus (HPV) infection which presents with solitary or multiple slightly elevated hyperkeratotic papules/plaques on soles. Due to plantar region's anatomical features, warts located in this area tend to ingrown. So far, HPV-1, −2, −3, −4, −27, −29, −57, −60, −63, −65, −66, and – 69 are isolated from verruca plantaris [61]. Although we can see tiny black dots which represent thrombosed, dilated capillaries on these hyperkeratotic papules with naked eye on occasion, in some cases it can not be seen and dermatoscopic examination is beneficial in these patients without paring the lesion. Lee el al. reported dermatoscopy of verruca plantaris as black and red dots on hyperkeratotic papilliform surface under polarized light [62].

4. Traumatic changes

4.1 Callus

Callus is localized hyperkeratosis of epidermis as a reaction of chronic irregular pressure or friction. It is mostly recognizable with naked eye, however in some cases clinicians have to make differential diagnosis between verruca and callus. Bae et al. showed homogenous opacity is diagnostic for callus and easily distinguishable from verruca under polarized light dermatoscopy [63].

4.2 Subcorneal hemorrhage

Subcorneal hemorrhage is a pigmented macule mainly located on palms and soles after trauma. By the reason of its similarity to acral melanocytic lesions and sometimes patient could not remember the history of trauma, it is important to

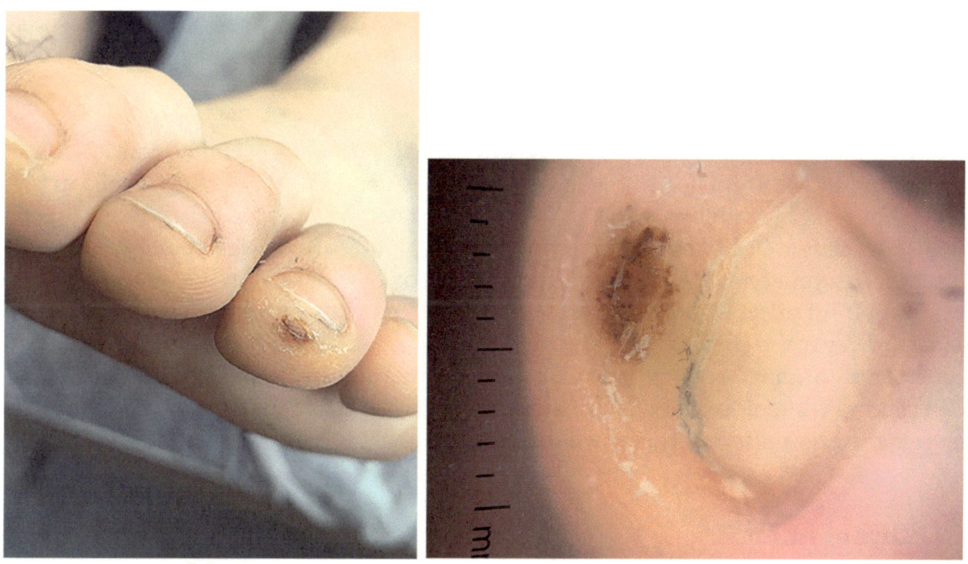

(a) (b)

Figure 8.
(a) Subcorneal hemorrhage. (b) Red-black satellite globules on a red-brown background.

distinguish. Complete or partial removal of pigmentation under scratch test is indicative for subcorneal hemorrhage. Zalaudek et al. reported sharp-dermarcated red-black homogeneous area with satellite globules in subcorneal hemorrhage [64]. **Figure 8a** shows subcorneal hemorrhage on toe and **Figure 8b** shows red-black satellite globules on a red-brown background.

5. Other diseases

5.1 Circumscribed palmar hypokeratosis

Circumscribed palmar hypokeratosis (CPH) is a rare epidermal malformation described by Perez in 2002 [65]. It is characterized by a localized reduction of the stratum corneum and typically presents as an isolated, well-circumscribed, atrophic, annular erythematous plaque with a slightly raised scaly border on the palmar surface, most commonly on the thenar or hypothenar eminence [66]. The exact mechanism of CPH is unknown, but it has been suggested that it may be due to local micro-trauma because of late onset and localization of lesions [66].

There are few studies in the literature describing the dermatoscopic findings of CPH. Ishiko et al. described that characteristic features of palmar hypokeratosis are stair-like desquamation and a homogeneous erythema with regularly distributed whitish spot (without jelly; erythema with stair-like desquamation with jelly; structureless erythema with regularly distributed whitish spots) [67]. Nishimura et al. confirmed stair-like desquamation and well-demarcated erythema scattered with white spots. They showed small reddish dots in the erythema that show the congestive capillaries in the papillary dermis [68].

Vilas Boas da Silva et al. showed dotted vessels over an erythematous background, along with and a vertical interruption and a moth-eaten profile in three women [66]. They also described the whitish streaks as another dermatoscopical finding of CPH for the first time [66]. It has been suggested that the white spots represent acrosyringium and correspond to marked hypokeratosis. The whitish streaks indicates furrows that are deeper on the hypothenar eminence. The reasons of the erythematous background might be the chronic inflammatory infiltrate, congestive capillaries, and thinned horny layer [68].

Considering the dermatoscopical and clinical findings of CPH, the main differential diagnoses are Bowen's disease and Mibelli porokeratosis. The characteristic dermatoscopical findings of Bowen's disease are clustered glomerular vessels, dry scales, small brown globules and structureless gray to brown pigmentation [66, 69]. Red spots shown in CPH may be confused with glomerular vessels seen in Bowen's disease. Asymmetric and clustered distribution of vessels seen in Bowen's disease can be helpful differentiating it from CPH. Porokeratosis shows a double rim of scale, however the characteristic stair-like desquamation rim is present in CPH. The central part of porokeratosis is usually hypopigmented and reveals dotted vessels. CPH shows white dots and whitish streaks which are not seen in porokeratosis may help in differentiating of these two diseases [66].

Conflict of interest

No conflict of interest.

Author details

Tubanur Çetinarslan[1*], Ece Gökyayla[2] and Aylin Türel Ermertcan[2]

1 Dermatology Clinic, Kırıkkale Yüksek İhtisas Hospital, Kırıkkale, Turkey

2 Department of Dermatology, Manisa Celal Bayar University, Manisa, Turkey

*Address all correspondence to: t_sarmis@windowslive.com

References

[1] Lallas A, Giacomel J, Argenziano G, et al. Dermoscopy in general dermatology: practical tips for the clinician. Br J Dermatol 2014; 170: 514-526.

[2] Çetinarslan T, Türel Ermertcan A, Temiz P. Dermoscopic clues of palmoplantar hyperkeratotic eczema and palmoplantar psoriasis: A prospective, comparative study of 90 patients. J Dermatol. 2020; 47(10): 1157-1165.

[3] Errichetti E, Stinco G. Dermoscopy in differential diagnosis of palmar psoriasis and chronic hand eczema. J Dermatol 2016; 43: 423-425.

[4] Yu X, Wei G, Shao C, et al. Analysis of dermoscopic characteristic for the differential diagnosis of palmoplantar psoriasis and palmoplantar eczema. Medicine (Baltimore) 2021; 100(5): e23828.

[5] Errichetti E, Stinco G. Dermoscopy in general dermatology: a practical overview. Dermatol Ther (Heidelb) 2016; 6: 471-507.

[6] Lallas A, Apalla Z, Argenziano G et al. Dermoscopic pattern of psoriatic lesions on specific body sites. Dermatology 2014; 228: 250– 254.

[7] Errichetti E, Lallas A, Di Stefani A, et al. Accuracy of dermoscopy in distinguishing erythroplasia of Queyrat from common forms of chronic balanitis: results from a multicentric observational study. J Eur Acad Dermatol Venereol. 2019; 33(5):966-972.

[8] Errichetti E, Stinco G. Comment on "Dermatoscopic features of lichen nitidus." Pediatr Dermatol. 2018; 35(6): 879-880.

[9] Vazquez-Lopez F, Kreusch J, Marghoob AA. Dermoscopic semiology: further insights into vascular features by screening a large spectrum of nontumoral skin lesions. Br J Dermatol 2004; 150:226-231.

[10] Errichetti E. Dermoscopy of Inflammatory Dermatoses (Inflam-moscopy): An Up-to-Date Overview. Dermatol Pract Concept. 2019; 9(3): 169-180.

[11] Boehncke WH, Schön MP. Psoriasis. Lancet. 2015; 386(9997):983-994.

[12] Farley E, Masrour S, McKey J, et al. Palmoplantar psoriasis: a phenotypical and clinical review with introduction of a new quality- of-life assessment tool. J Am Acad Dermatol 2009; 60: 1024-1031.

[13] Griffiths CE, Christophers E, Barker JN, et al. A classification of psoriasis vulgaris according to phenotype. Br J Dermatol 2007; 156:258-262.

[14] Misiak-Galazka M, Wolska H, Rudnicka L. What do we know about palmoplantar pustulosis?. J Eur Acad Dermatol Venereol 2017; 31: 38-44.

[15] Errichetti E, Stinco G. The practical usefulness of dermoscopy in general dermatology. G Ital Dermatol Venereol. 2015; 150(5):533-546.

[16] Zalaudek I, Argenziano G, Di Stefani A, et al. Dermoscopy in general dermatology. Dermatology 2006; 212: 7-18.

[17] Vazquez-Lopez F, Manjon-Haces JA, Maldonado-Seral C, et al. Dermoscopic features of plaque psoriasis and lichen planus: new observations. Dermatology 2003; 207: 151-156.

[18] Errichetti E, Lacarrubba F, Micali G, et al. Differentiation of pityriasis lichenoides chronica from guttate psoriasis by dermoscopy. Clin Exp Dermatol 2015; 40: 804-806.

[19] Vazquez-Lopez F, Zaballos P, Fueyo-Casado A, et al. A dermoscopy subpattern of plaque-type psoriasis: red globular rings. Arch Dermatol 2007; 143: 1612.

[20] Lacarrubba F, Pellacani G, Gurgone S, et al. Advances in non-invasive techniques as aids to the diagnosis and monitoring of therapeutic response in plaque psoriasis: a review. Int J Dermatol 2015; 54: 626-634.

[21] Micali G, Nardone B, Scuderi A, et al. Videodermatoscopy enhances diagnostic capability in some forms of palmar and/or plantar psoriasis. Am J Clin Dermatol 2008; 9: 119-122.

[22] Lallas A, Kyrgidis A, Tzellos TG, et al. Accuracy of dermoscopic criteria for the diagnosis of psoriasis, dermatitis, lichen planus and pityriasis rosea. Br J Dermatol 2012; 166: 1198-1205.

[23] Lallas A, Zalaudek I, Argenziano G, et al. Dermoscopy in general dermatology. Dermatol Clin 2013; 31: 679-694.

[24] Calonje JE, Brenn T, Lazar AJF, et al. Spongiotic, psoriasiform and pustular dermatoses. In: Calonje JE, Brenn T, Lazar AJF, McKee PH, eds. McKees Pathology of the Skin, 4th edn. Philadelphia, PA: Elsevier Saunders: 2012. p. 183-184.

[25] Errichetti E, Stinco G. Dermoscopy as a supportive instrument in the differentiation of the main types of acquired keratoderma due to dermatological disorders. J Eur Acad Dermatol Venereol. 2016; 30(12): 229-231.

[26] Calonje E, Neill S, Bunker C, et al. Diseases of the anogenital skin. In: Calonje E, Brenn T, Lazar A, et al. (eds) McKee's pathology of the skin, 4th ed. Edinburgh, United Kingdom: Elsevier Saunders, 2012. p. 465-472.

[27] Errichetti E, Stinco G. Dermoscopy in differentiating palmar syphiloderm from palmar papular psoriasis. Int J STD AIDS. 2017; 28(14): 1461-1463.

[28] Mrowietz U. Pustular eruptions of palms and soles. In: Goldsmith, ed. Fitzpatrick's Dermatology in General Medicine. New York: McGraw-Hill; 2012. p. 252-259.

[29] Meier M, Sheth PB. Clinical spectrum and severity of psoriasis. Curr Probl Dermatol. 2009; 38:1-20.

[30] Lallas A, Errichetti E. Papulosquamous disorders. In: Lallas A, Errichetti E, Ioannides D, eds. Dermatoscopy in General Dermatology. Boca Raton, FL: CRC Press; 2018. p. 2-51

[31] Errichetti E, Pegolo E, Stinco G. Dermatoscopy as an auxiliary tool in the early differential diagnosis of acute generalized exanthematous pustulosis (AGEP) and exanthematous (morbilliform) drug eruption. J Am Acad Dermatol 2016; 74: 29-31.

[32] Errichetti E, Stinco G. Dermatoscopy in life-threatening and severe acute rashes. Clin Dermatol. 2020; 38(1): 113-121.

[33] M. Uehara, S. Ofuji, The morphogenesis of pustulosis palmaris et plantaris, Arch. Dermatol. 1974; 109 (4): 518-520.

[34] Hersle K, Mobacken H. Hyperkeratotic dermatitis of the palms. Br J Dermatol. 1982; 107: 195-202.

[35] Errichetti E, Piccirillo A, Stinco G. Dermoscopy as an auxiliary tool in the differentiation of the main types of erythroderma due to dermatological disorders. Int J Dermatol 2016; 55: 616-618.

[36] Braun-Falco M. Hereditary palmoplantar keratodermas. J Dtsch Dermatol Ges 2009; 7: 971-984; quiz 84-5.

[37] Schiller S, Seebode C, Hennies HC, et al. Palmoplantar keratoderma (PPK): acquired and genetic causes of a not so rare disease. JDDG: Journal Der Deutschen Dermatologischen Gesellschaft 2014; 12(9): 781-788.

[38] Roenneberg S, Biedermann T. Pityriasis rubra pilaris: algorithms for diagnosis and treatment. J Eur Acad Dermatol Venereol. 2018; 32(6): 889-898.

[39] Giordano LMC, De la Fuente LA, Lorca JMB, et al. Tinea nigra: Report of three pediatrics cases. Rev Chil Pediatr. 2018; 89(4): 506-510.

[40] Aram H, Zeidenbaum M. Palmo-plantar hyperkeratosis in mycosis fungoides. J Am Acad Dermatol 1985; 13: 897-899.

[41] Elewski BE, Greer DL. Hendersonula toruloidea and Scytalidium hyalinum. Review and update. Arch Dermatol. 1991; 127(7): 1041-1044.

[42] Goodlad J, Calonje E. Cutaneous lymphoproliferative diseases and related disorders. In: Calonje JE, Brenn T, Lazar AJF, McKee PH, eds. McKee's Pathology of the Skin, 4th edn. Elsevier Saunders, Philadelphia, 2012. p. 1313-1340.

[43] Yan AC, Aasi SZ, Alms WJ, et al. Aquagenic palmoplantar keratoderma. J Am Acad Dermatol 2001; 44: 696-699.

[44] Fernández-Crehuet P, Ruiz-Villaverde R. Dermoscopic features of aquagenic syringeal acrokeratoderma. Int J Dermatol. 2016; 55(7): 407-408.

[45] Sezer E, Erkek E, Duman D, et al. Dermatoscopy as an adjunctive diagnostic tool in aquagenic syringeal acrokeratoderma. Dermatology. 2012; 225(2): 97-99.

[46] Lacarrubba F, Verzì AE, Leonardi S, et al. Palmar wrinkling: Identification of a peculiar pattern at incident light dermoscopy with confocal microscopy correlation. J Am Acad Dermatol. 2016; 75(4): 143-145.

[47] Landis M, Bohyer C, Bahrami S, et al. Palmoplantar lichen planus: A rare presentation of a common disease. J Dermatol Case Rep. 2008; 2:8-10.

[48] James WD, Elston DM, Berger TG. Clinical Dermatology. 11th ed. United Kingdom: Saunders Elsevier; 2011. p. 222-223.

[49] Park SH, Kim SW, Noh TW, et al. A Case of Palmar Lichen Nitidus Presenting as a Clinical Feature of Pompholyx. Ann Dermatol. 2010; 22: 235-237.

[50] Qian G, Wang H, Wu J, et al. Different dermoscopic patterns of palmoplantar and nonpalmoplantar lichen nitidus. J Am Acad Dermatol. 2015; 73(3): 101-103.

[51] Errichetti E, Stinco G. Dermoscopy in tinea manuum. An Bras Dermatol. 2018; 93(3): 447-448.

[52] Jakhar D, Kaur I, Sonthalia S. Dermoscopy of Tinea Manuum. Indian Dermatol Online J. 2019; 10(2): 210-211.

[53] Cabo H. Dermatoscopia, Segunda edición, Buenos Aires 2016, Ediciones Journal, 14 p. 328.

[54] Navarrete M, Castillo A, Sánchez A, et al. Dermatología CMQ 2012; 10(3): 205-211.

[55] Guarenti IM, Almeida HL Jr, Leitão AH, et al. Scanning electron microscopy of tinea nigra. An Bras Dermatol. 2014; 89(2): 334-336.

[56] Noguchi H, Hiruma M, Inoue Y, et al. Tinea nigra showing a parallel ridge pattern on dermoscopy. J Dermatol 2015; 42: 1-3.

[57] Nazzaro G, Ponziani A, Cavicchini S. Tinea nigra: A diagnostic pitfall. J Am Acad Dermatol 2016; 75: 219-220.

[58] Tognetti L, Sbano P, Fimiani M, et al. Dermoscopy of Biett's sign and differential diagnosis with annular maculo-papular rashes with scaling. Indian J Dermatol Venereol Leprol 2017; 83: 270-273.

[59] Bristow IR, Lee YL. Pitted keratolysis: a clinical review. J Am Podiatr Med Assoc. 2014; 104(2): 177-182.

[60] Lockwood LL, Gehrke S, Navarini AA. Dermoscopy of Pitted Keratolysis. Case Rep Dermatol. 2010; 2(2):146-148.

[61] Witchey DJ, Witchey NB, Roth-Kauffman MM, et al. Plantar Warts: Epidemiology, Pathophysiology, and Clinical Management. J Am Osteopath Assoc. 2018; 118(2):92-105.

[62] Lee DY, Park JH, Lee JH, et al. The use of dermoscopy for the diagnosis of plantar wart. J Eur Acad Dermatol Venereol. 2009;23(6): 726-727.

[63] Bae JM, Kang H, Kim HO, et al. Differential diagnosis of plantar wart from corn, callus and healed wart with the aid of dermoscopy. Br J Dermatol. 2009;160(1): 220-222.

[64] Zalaudek I, Argenziano G, Soyer HP, et al. Dermoscopy of subcorneal hematoma. Dermatol Surg. 2004;30(9): 1229-1232.

[65] Perez A, Rütten A, Gold R, et al. Circumscribed palmar or plantar hypokeratosis: a distinctive epidermal malformation of the palms or soles. J Am Acad Dermatol. 2002; 47: 21-27.

[66] Vilas Boas da Silva PT, Rodríguez-Lomba E, Avilés-Izquierdo JA, et al. Dermoscopic features of circumscribed palmar hypokeratosis. JAMA Dermatol 2017; 153: 609-611.

[67] Ishiko A, Dekio I, Fujimoto A, et al. Abnormal keratin expression in circumscribed palmar hypokeratosis. J Am Acad Dermatol. 2007; 57(2): 285-291.

[68] Nishimura M, Nishie W, Nakazato S, et al. Circumscribed palmar hypokeratosis: correlation between histopathological patterns and dermoscopic findings. Br J Dermatol. 2012; 167(1): 221-222.

[69] Lallas A, Errichetti E. Miscellaneous inflammatory diseases. In: Lallas A, Errichetti E, Ioannides D, editors. Dermoscopy in General Dermatology. 1st ed. Boca Raton: CRC; 2018. p. 134.

Chapter 7

Precautions on Contact Dermatoscopy and Other Practices in the Pandemic of COVID-19

Walid Al-Zyoud and Dana Erekat

Abstract

In the age of the pandemic of COVID-19, there is a considerable need for hospitals that triggers many challenges for health care providers to keep themselves and their patients protected from any nosocomial infections, including viral, fungal and bacterial infections. Among health care providers, dermatologists play a vital role in performing dermatoscopy free from *Staphylococcus epidermidis*, *Micrococcus*, and *Corynebacterium* species reported to be identified on the dermoscopic lenses and their adaptors. There is also a possibility for SARS-CoV-2, a member of coronaviruses, to be transmissible from patient to a physician or vice versa or even from a physician to one of her or his family members. SARS-CoV-2 can be transferred through the mucus membranes of the human eyes. This chapter will flag the importance of having a detailed list of precautions for dermatologists and patients to make clinical practice as safe as possible.

Keywords: dermatoscopy, COVID-19, nosocomial, precautions, dermatology

1. Introduction

The novel coronavirus (SARS-CoV-2 or 2019-nCoV) originated in Wuhan, China, in December 2019 and caused deadly acute respiratory syndrome and hence the pandemic COVID-19 [1] with an exponential increase in the number of infected persons. It is well-known that the pandemic of COVID-19 has affected everyone and every sector we are involved in, either physically mentally or even economically. One of the most affected sectors is the sector of public health. The health care providers represent the front line defence and the most critical components of any healthcare system across the globe. The pandemic of COVID-19 has put an unprecedented challenge on the healthcare providers, including dermatologists [2, 3] to cope with such an outbreak. Many studies have reported that SARS-CoV-2 can stay on inanimate surfaces such as stainless steel, copper, plastics, and papers [4–6]. Our contact with lifeless surfaces might represent a source of infection if we contact a living tissue or mucus of suspected or confirmed cases of COVID-19; this was our motivation to write this chapter to summarise precautions from the literature on how dermatologists can apply some contact practices when dealing with expected infections. This chapter has been divided into five sections: the first section of the introduction; section two about consent and precaution; section three about aesthetic procedure protection, section four about general principles, and the last section about dermatoscopy procedures. The chapter references focused on the published expertise of the prestigious Indian Association of Dermatologists Venereologists and Leprologists (IADVL) and the World Health Organisation (WHO) in this field.

2. Consent and precaution

The dermatologist and patient should consider the precautions of the COVID-19 pandemic. A dermatologist's ability to manage their patients care is the single most critical criterion for patient safety. Depending on the type of treatment being conducted, the risk-benefit ratio of undergoing a procedure should be considered. Procedures that need many appointments to the institution for follow-up are best postponed, so performing treatments requiring the least number of sessions is preferable [7]. Patients should be aware of the possibility of being exposed to the infection on their visit to the healthcare facility. It is better if the dermatologist explains the risk of invasiveness of the treatment and contracting the virus. The dermatologist may also list the side effects of the procedure that may need counselling pre-procedure. Patients on treatment after the pandemic may need to be monitored by video teleconsultation serial imaging, or followed up with a USB or portable patient-friendly dermatoscope, while some other patients starting treatments may still need to undergo onsite visits and procedures [7].

It was proven that even vaccinated individuals can get infected with COVID-19 [8]. If any staff member tests positive or expresses symptoms of infection, the personnel should undergo screen testing with Polymerase Chain Reaction (PCR). According to the Centers of Disease Control (CDC) in the United States of America, the individual with a positive result should remain in quarantine until testing negative after 5 to 7 days if the individual is fully vaccinated and after 14 days if not fully vaccinated to prevent the spread of the virus [9]. Rotational shifts of staff members, in which staff members are divided into two teams for 7 days on-duty and 7 days off-duty, might be a viable alternative [10].

It is essential to support medical staff mentally during the pandemic and on the other hand avoid frightening the patients in an excessive way so that they do not abstain from medically justified procedures, including skin cancer surgery. Some individuals might seek counselling sessions and therapy to stay in their best mind and energy through the tough times. This allows the staff to stay more balanced about the seriousness of the virus.

2.1 Waiting, consultation, and operating rooms precaution

Disposable masks and sanitizers should be offered to the patients at the entrance of the healthcare institute, as all patients should enter with three layered or cotton masks. Gloves can be provided as extra protection to avoid direct skin contact with surfaces that may be exposed to the virus. A thermometer should be used at the entrance to measure the fever of individuals before entering the facility, as high fever can be a sign of infection. The waiting rooms should adhere to social distancing, with 2 meters (~6 feet) distance between individuals [11]. To avoid overcrowding, patients are allowed to have one or even no companion with them to the appointment. The waiting room should be made only available for individuals who come in time for their appointments. If a person is late, the appointment should be rescheduled for another time. The patient should be transferred promptly to the consultation room without waiting long in the waiting area, and social distance is essential even if a close inspection is required during counselling [10].

The staff must disinfect all devices and tools that come in contact with the patient. The operating rooms must be sterilised after each patient [12]. To avoid contact with

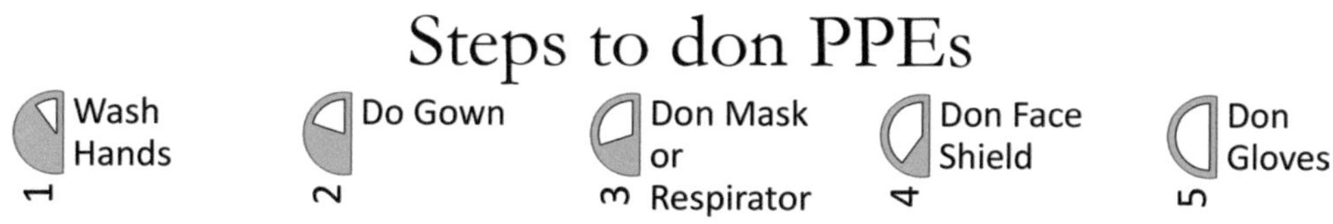
Steps to don PPEs
1 Wash Hands
2 Do Gown
3 Don Mask or Respirator
4 Don Face Shield
5 Don Gloves

Figure 1.
Steps to put on PPEs, including gown.

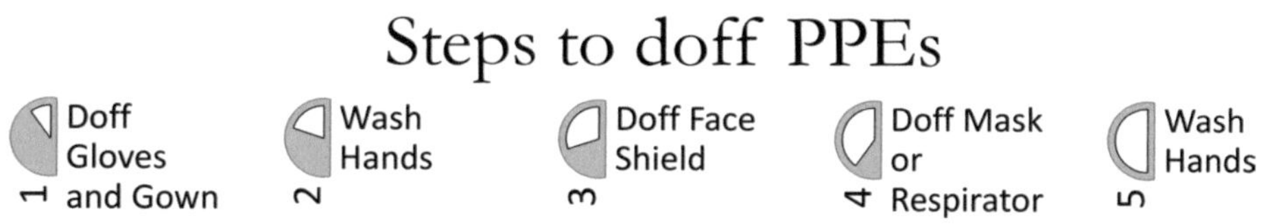
Steps to doff PPEs
1 Doff Gloves and Gown
2 Wash Hands
3 Doff Face Shield
4 Doff Mask or Respirator
5 Wash Hands

Figure 2.
Steps to take off PPEs, including gown.

numerous surfaces throughout the process, the patient should be required to wear a gown or overall. To disinfect the operating rooms, remove all machines, beds, stools, and chairs from the room and spray a sodium hypochlorite solution over all surfaces, including the floor, doors, windows, curtains, and cupboards [10]. The operating rooms should have ventilation and enhanced airflow. A powerful exhaust fan can be used in the operation area to optimise airflow, with stand-alone air conditioning devices in the rooms instead of the central air conditioning system [10].

2.2 Personalised protective equipment (PPE)

PPEs are protective equipment meant to protect employees' health by limiting their exposure to viruses. Goggles, face shields, masks, gloves, coveralls/gowns (with or without aprons), head cover, and shoe covers are all examples of PPE. It is advised for all the staff in the clinic to use PPE for extra protection from the virus. The PPE kit differs depending on the procedure and an individual's risk of exposure.

Gown, mask, goggles/face shield, then gloves are the steps in the PPEs donning sequence, whereas gloves, goggles/face shield, gown, mask, then hand hygiene or gown and gloves, goggles/face shield, mask, and lastly, hand hygiene are the steps in the PPEs doffing sequence (**Figures 1** and **2**). Hand hygiene should be conducted before going on to the next stage if hands contact any contaminated PPE surface. They should be disposed of accordingly, depending on the procedure. The interior of the biohazard bag should be treated with a 1 per cent sodium hypochlorite solution before being knotted, and the exterior should be decontaminated with 1 per cent sodium hypochlorite [10].

The N-95 masks can be used multiple times if disinfected correctly. The authors in the reference below suggest that masks can be discarded after five usages. After use, place the mask in a permeable paper mask and set it aside for 4 days to dry. On day 6, it should be used again. Similarly, vaporised hydrogen peroxide and U.V. germicidal radiation (UVC 254 nm) can also be used to decontaminate the N-95 masks [10].

3. Aesthetic procedure protection

The aesthetic procedures are classified into three categories depending on the invasiveness of the procedure; these categories are invasive, minimally invasive, and non-invasive. According to the Indian Association of Dermatologists Venereologists

Invasive	Minimally Invasive	Non-Invasive
• Goggles	• Goggles	• N-95 respirator mask
• Face-shield	• N-95 respirator mask	• Latex/nitrile gloves
• N-95 respirator mask	• Latex/nitrile gloves	
• Surgical gloves	• Gown	
• Gown		
• Head cover		
• Shoe cover		

Table 1.
Protection and precautions of the aesthetic procedures to be utilised.

and Leprologists (IADVL) each category requires different protection and precautions [7] summarised in **Table 1**. Invasive procedures include those that have the potential for aerosolisation and ablation because they expose the patient and health workers to the infection [7]. It is advised only to perform invasive procedures if no other treatment is possible. The non-invasive procedures require basic protection and caution. The dermatologist should wear a N-95 respirator mask and Latex/Nitrile gloves. The patient is required to wear a three-layered mask. In contrast, the precautions of minimally invasive procedures include advanced caution, moderate protection, and additional protective equipment. Reasonable protection includes goggles, a N-95 respirator mask, Latex/Nitrile gloves, and a gown. Extreme caution, advanced safety, and additional protective equipment are mandatory to perform invasive procedures. Advanced protection requires goggles, face-shield, N-95 respirator mask, surgical gloves, coverall/gowns, head cover, and shoe cover.

4. General principles

The World Health Organisation (WHO) have issued a list of precautions and recommendations guideline to help prevent the spread of COVID-19. The facility must follow these guidelines for the safety of both the patients and staff. Personalised protective equipment (PPE) should be worn with an examination in negative pressure rooms must be followed if there is a high possibility of being exposed to infection [12].

1. All procedures should occur in a ventilated area, with the required protection used depending on the procedure.

2. Some patients may have an asymptomatic syndrome, so everyone should adhere to social distancing and universal precautions (WHO).

3. The instruments and tools in the facility should be sanitised with different chemicals depending on the type of material; this applies to dermatoscopes.

4. The tools should be sterilised, and the region that will be examined should be disinfected before starting the procedure.

5. Replace medical tools and products with disposables if available.

6. Tools and materials used in the examination or the procedure should be disposed of as per biomedical waste guidelines, and all surfaces must be cleaned with 60–90% isopropyl alcohol.

7. Disposable bins should be available in all rooms.

8. Patients should wear a mask at all times to prevent the spread of infection unless the treated area is around the mouth and nose.

9. Immunosuppressed patients and those on immunosuppressive medication should avert invasive procedures [7].

10. Procedures can be performed safely if an individual is on a regular hydroxy-chloroquine dose for rheumatoid arthritis patients or if an individual is on COVID-19 prophylaxis protocol [7].

4.1 Avoided procedures

Some treatment procedures might have a high risk of exposure to infection; hence, safer alternative treatments can be used instead of what is needed to be avoided. For example, platelet-rich plasma, platelet-rich factor, and growth factor concentrate are part of the blood and blood product treatments that can be avoided until after the pandemic, while mesotherapy using hair growth concentrates can substitute these procedures. If medical facials are not essential, they should be deferred and alternated with a prescription from the dermatologist. Carbon facials are avoided because they are plume generating procedures that need extreme caution [7]. Procedures such as laser toning and carbon peels can be postponed or performed with proper PPE/overalls and the use of disposable equipment [10]. The carbon peel, just like the carbon facials, highly generates plumes.

It is obligatory to use a complete COVID-19 PPE kit for dermabrasion procedures; otherwise, they should be postponed. All disposable and personal protection kits should be discarded accordingly. Fat grafting procedures must be deferred because the danger of transmission is serious while handling tissues [7]. Hyaluronic acid filler can be used instead. It is best to avoid hot probe electrosurgery procedures that produce plumes. These procedures are electrofulguration, electrodessication, and electrocautery. To limit plume generation, cold probe devices such as higher frequency—radiofrequency devices may be utilised for electro sectioning [7]. Avoiding various procedures such as cosmetic tattooing, tattoo removing and dermaplaning is recommended. Mucosal and oozy/fissured lesions should be deferred in dermatoscopy [12].

4.2 Recommendations for specific procedures

Some procedures may need particular recommendations for precaution against the virus.

1. Fillers, toxins, threads, and lipolysis injections are classified under injectables. For safety, the dermatologist should follow basic protection and caution. Use povidone-iodine to cover oral and nasal mucosa for procedures around the nose and perioral region since it has been found to be viricidal against SARSCoV2 for 3 h [13]. SteristripsTM or an appropriate skin dressing should be worn for 48 h after the surgery, followed by antibiotic cream and medical plaster within the first 2 days [7].

2. In micro-needling, use disposable derma rollers, discard the cartridge of motorised devices, and sterilise the tip of radiofrequency devices using glutaraldehyde after each patient [14].

3. Non-invasive and minimally invasive chemical peels for face, nail, and body need prescribed skin barrier repair creams after treatment. In the post-care recommendations, the patient should be urged to moisturise well since dry skin after a peel might lead to more frequent touching of the face and the theoretical risk of virus transmission through abraded skin.

4. Dermabrasions are better avoided, while microdermabrasion can be done with extreme care because dry skin scrubbing can cause aerosol generation.

5. Use moderate protection for procedures that require radiofrequency for extra precaution.

6. Nonsurgical body contouring procedures require basic protection and caution as they are not dangerous to perform.

7. The dermatologist should use 60–90% isopropyl alcohol swaps to clean the scoped lesion with alcohol-containing solutions utilised as interface medium in dermatoscopy. Instead of the handheld contact dermatoscope, noncontact polarised dermatoscope, video, or USB dermatoscopy can be used [12].

8. Most various procedures are safe. Electroporation, skin boosters, and low light laser therapy are non-invasive or minimally invasive procedures that require almost no pre-or- post-care. Because microblading can cause some bleeding, it is advised to use full PPE and apply sterile/Tegaderm™ [7] wound dressing overnight to ensure skin closure.

9. In laser and energy-based devices, the lens of the machines is cleaned with 70% ethyl alcohol [10]. Special PPE kits are worn while performing carbon laser peels, ablative lasers, fractional resurfacing, tattoo removal, IPL photorejuvenation, mono/bi/multipolar radio frequency (RF) firming, and High intensity Focused Ultrasound (HiFU) [10]. Disposable cup and brush for carbon solution or cooling gel application and disposable cling wrapping for the handpiece and machine and cooling equipment disinfection can be used when needed. Different treatments require particular caution and protection depending on the technology used; please see **Table 2** below.

Technique	**Technology**
Carbon laser peel	Q-switched Nd:YAG laser
Ablative lasers	Continuous wave CO_2 laser
Laser epilation	810 nm, 1064 nm, 755 nm, or triple wavelength
Fractional resurfacing	CO_2, Er:YAG, Er:glass, thulium laser
IPL photo rejuvenation, mono/bi/multipolar RF firming, HiFU	IPL, mono/bipolar RF, HiFU
Tattoo removal	Nanosecond Q switched Nd:YAG, HiFU or picosecond laser

IPL: intense pulsed light; HiFU: high intensity focused ultrasound; RF: radio frequency; Q-switched laser: Quality-switched laser; Nd:YAG laser: (neodymium-doped yttrium aluminium garnet laser; Nd:$Y_3Al_5O_{12}$); Er:YAG laser: (erbium-doped yttrium aluminium garnet laser); Er:glass laser: erbium glass lasers.

Table 2.
The technology of laser and energy based procedures [10].

5. Dermatoscopy procedures

The dermatologist should follow basic protection and caution before performing procedures. There must be smoke evacuators and ventilation in all the rooms where the procedures are performed as some procedures may generate plume. The dermatoscope should be wiped with 70% isopropyl alcohol and covered with a disposable dermoscopic lens [12].

These precautions may decrease the possibility of virus transmission through the device. Between the dermatoscope lens and the lesion, a polyvinyl chloride (PVC) film is applied, and a transparent adhesive tape can be put to aid contact dermatoscopy once the immersion fluid has been deposited with a glass slide can be placed over the lesion in front of the dermatoscope [12]. The PCV, tape, and glass slide act as a barrier between the patient and the device. For microscopy, a disposable polyethylene tube can be used with a USB dermatoscope [12]. It is recommended that if the dermatologist is going to use mobile phone to see photos with a dermatoscope to clean it first. A digital dermatoscopy report is preferred because an audiovisual paperless communication is desirable specially when there is a distance between the patients and the healthcare providers. Some limitation of digital dermatoscopy may remain, such as low resolution images, ethical dilemma, patient's privacy and medico-legal responsibility.

All dermoscopic examination materials should be disposed of according to biomedical waste rules. To decrease the nosocomial infection when practicing dermatoscopy, there are many precautions to be taken into consideration, especially when dealing with suspected COVID-19 cases such as:

1. Telephone and or web-based interview form to be filled before dermatoscopy to check the travel history and the presence of any symptoms [10]. This form should include instructions for patients on the clinic's measures related to coronavirus.

2. To use commercially available and disposable dermoscopic lens cover.

3. To use transparent adhesive tapes or microscopic glass slides over the skin lesions when contact dermatoscopy is applied [15].

6. Conclusion

It is vital to have a set of precautions and recommendations for the dermatologists to help them carry on their clinical practice safely in COVID-19 era; it is rightly said that "prevention is better than cure". The pandemic of COVID-19 has significantly affected many sectors all over the world. We did not expect such a catastrophic outbreak, and it might not be the last. The presence of clear and informative safety consensus guidelines for the dermatologists when dealing with suspected or confirmed cases of COVID-19 is essential to stop the viral transmission from the patients to health care providers and then to their family members.

Acknowledgements

The authors thank Mr. Josip Knapic, the author service manager at Intechopen Limited (U.K.), for following up during this chapter's writing phase.

Conflict of interest

The authors declare no conflict of interest.

Author details

Walid Al-Zyoud* and Dana Erekat
German Jordanian University, Amman, Jordan

*Address all correspondence to: walid.alzyoud@gju.edu.jo

References

[1] Zhu N, Zhang D, Wang W, Li X, Yang B, Song J, et al. A novel coronavirus from patients with pneumonia in China, 2019. The New England Journal of Medicine. 2020;**382**:727-733. DOI: 10.1056/NEJMOA2001017

[2] Bai Y, Yao L, Wei T, Tian F, Jin DY, Chen L, et al. Presumed asymptomatic carrier transmission of COVID-19. Journal of the American Medical Association. 2020;**323**:1406-1407. DOI: 10.1001/JAMA.2020.2565

[3] Piccolo V, Argenziano G. The impact of novel coronavirus on dermatology. Dermatology Practical & Conceptual. 2020;**10**(2):e2020049. DOI: 10.5826/DPC.1002A49

[4] Kampf G, Todt D, Pfaender S, Steinmann E. Persistence of coronaviruses on inanimate surfaces and their inactivation with biocidal agents. The Journal of Hospital Infection. 2020;**104**:246-251. DOI: 10.1016/J.JHIN.2020.01.022

[5] Belluco S, Mancin M, Marzoli F, Bortolami A, Mazzetto E, Pezzuto A, et al. Prevalence of SARS-CoV-2 RNA on inanimate surfaces: A systematic review and meta-analysis. European Journal of Epidemiology. 2021;**36**:685-707. DOI: 10.1007/S10654-021-00784-Y

[6] Piana A, Colucci ME, Valeriani F, Marcolongo A, Sotgiu G, Pasquarella C, et al. Monitoring COVID-19 transmission risks by quantitative real-time PCR tracing of droplets in hospital and living environments. MSphere. 2021;**6**(1):e01070-20. DOI: 10.1128/MSPHERE.01070-20

[7] Arora G, Arora S, Talathi A, Kandhari R, Joshi V, Langar S, et al. Safer practice of aesthetic dermatology during the COVID-19 pandemic: Recommendations by SIG aesthetics (IADVL Academy). Indian Dermatology Online Journal. 2020;**11**:534. DOI: 10.4103/IDOJ.IDOJ_328_20

[8] Antonelli M, Penfold RS, Merino J, Sudre CH, Molteni E, Berry S, et al. Risk factors and disease profile of post-vaccination SARS-CoV-2 infection in UK users of the COVID symptom study app: A prospective, community-based, nested, case-control study. The Lancet Infectious Diseases. 2021:1. DOI: 10.1016/S1473-3099(21)00460-6

[9] COVID-19 Quarantine and Isolation. CDC. 2021. Available from: https://www.cdc.gov/coronavirus/2019-ncov/your-health/quarantine-isolation.html [Accessed: December 10, 2021]

[10] Dhawan S, Kumari P, De A, Pall A, Pudukadan D, Romi E, et al. Lasers use in dermatology practice in the evolving COVID-19 scenario: Recommendations by SIG Lasers (IADVL Academy). Indian Dermatology Online Journal. 2020;**11**:337. DOI: 10.4103/IDOJ.IDOJ_239_20

[11] Prevent Getting Sick. CDC. 2021. Available from: https://www.cdc.gov/coronavirus/2019-ncov/prevent-getting-sick/index.html [Accessed: December 10, 2021]

[12] Jakhar D, Bhat YJ, Chatterjee M, Keshavmurthy V, Ankad BS, Jha AK, et al. Dermoscopy practice during COVID-19 pandemic: Recommendations by SIG dermoscopy (IADVL Academy). Indian Dermatology Online Journal. 2020;**11**: 343. DOI: 10.4103/IDOJ.IDOJ_231_20

[13] Bali RK, Chaudhry K. Maxillofacial surgery and COVID-19, The Pandemic!! Journal of Oral and Maxillofacial Surgery. 2020;**19**:159. DOI: 10.1007/S12663-020-01361-8

[14] Sharad M. Standard guidelines for electrosurgery with radiofrequency current. Indian Journal of Dermatology,

Venereology and Leprology. 2009;**75**:83-89. Available from: https://ijdvl.com/standard-guidelines-for-electrosurgery-with-radiofrequency-current/ [Accessed: November 19, 2021]

[15] Mun J-H, Park S-M, Ko H-C, Kim B-S, Kim M-B. Prevention of possible cross-infection among patients by dermoscopy: A brief review of the literature and our suggestion. Dermatology Practical & Conceptual. 2013;**3**(4):7. DOI: 10.5826/DPC.0304A07